Technology in Hospitals

Studies in Social Economics

TITLES PUBLISHED

STUDIES IN SOCIAL ECONOMICS

Louise B. Russell

Technology in Hospitals: Medical Advances and Their Diffusion

THE BROOKINGS INSTITUTION
Washington, D.C.

Copyright © 1979 by
THE BROOKINGS INSTITUTION
1775 Massachusetts Avenue, N.W., Washington, D.C. 20036

Library of Congress Cataloging in Publication Data:
Russell, Louise B
    Technology in hospitals.
    (Studies in social economics)
    Includes index.
    1. Hospitals—Furniture, equipment, etc.
2. Hospitals—United States—Furniture, equipment,
etc. 3. Medical innovations—United States.
4. Diffusion of innovations—United States.
5. Hospitals—United States—Cost of operation.
I. Title. II. Series. [DNLM: 1. Technology,
Medical.   2. Equipment and supplies, Hospital.
3. Hospital departments.   4. Hospital units.
WX147 R964t]
RA968.R8   362.1'1'028   79-10737
ISBN 0-8157-7630-6
ISBN 0-8157-7629-2 pbk.

9 8 7 6 5 4 3 2 1

THE BROOKINGS INSTITUTION is an independent organization devoted to nonpartisan research, education, and publication in economics, government, foreign policy, and the social sciences generally. Its principal purposes are to aid in the development of sound public policies and to promote public understanding of issues of national importance.

The Institution was founded on December 8, 1927, to merge the activities of the Institute for Government Research, founded in 1916, the Institute of Economics, founded in 1922, and the Robert Brookings Graduate School of Economics and Government, founded in 1924.

The Board of Trustees is responsible for the general administration of the Institution, while the immediate direction of the policies, program, and staff is vested in the President, assisted by an advisory committee of the officers and staff. The by-laws of the Institution state: "It is the function of the Trustees to make possible the conduct of scientific research, and publication, under the most favorable conditions, and to safeguard the independence of the research staff in the pursuit of their studies and in the publication of the results of such studies. It is not a part of their function to determine, control, or influence the conduct of particular investigations or the conclusions reached."

The President bears final responsibility for the decision to publish a manuscript as a Brookings book. In reaching his judgment on the competence, accuracy, and objectivity of each study, the President is advised by the director of the appropriate research program and weighs the views of a panel of expert outside readers who report to him in confidence on the quality of the work. Publication of a work signifies that it is deemed a competent treatment worthy of public consideration but does not imply endorsement of conclusions or recommendations.

The Institution maintains its position of neutrality on issues of public policy in order to safeguard the intellectual freedom of the staff. Hence interpretations or conclusions in Brookings publications should be understood to be solely those of the authors and should not be attributed to the Institution, to its trustees, officers, or other staff members, or to the organizations that support its research.

Foreword

New techniques and new technologies have wrought major changes in hospital practice in the last several decades. Intensive care units, renal dialysis, open-heart surgery, and many other innovations have been part of the revolution in what hospitals can provide and in what the public expects. But they have been a mixed blessing: technology has come in for a good deal of blame as a major contributor to the rapid increase in hospital costs, especially over the last decade.

This study examines the recent history of technological diffusion in hospitals and considers some of the new technologies in detail. Its conclusion is that technological changes are not the true cause of rising costs The problem lies with the humane desire to see that no one has to forgo medical care because of its cost—to see that needed care is provided. The growth of private insurance and the introduction of Medicare and Medicaid are the practical manifestations of that desire.

But the endless list of things that could and should be done in medical care could easily absorb most of the nation's resources. In the author's view, stemming the rise in costs does not await new methods of budgeting and reimbursement, but rather requires that costs be considered even when health is at stake. When the problem is put this way, it becomes clear that restraining costs is likely to be so politically difficult and painful that the nation may well choose to continue present policies rather than restrict access to medical care.

The author is grateful to Margaret Windus and Carole Kitti of the National Science Foundation for their encouragement during the course of the research. She is also grateful to Charles Sanders, William Gould, Rashi Fein, and Uwe Reinhardt for reading and commenting on the manuscript. A great many people in government and private organizations—too many to list—deserve thanks for helping track down the data needed for the study. For help in the collection of information about policies in other countries the author is indebted to Vicente Navarro (all countries), Simone Sandier and C. Dutreil (France), David Kinnersley and Clifford Graham (United Kingdom), and Gunnar Wennström and Egon Jonsson (Sweden).

Carol Burke helped the author with the research and writing of an earlier report that formed the basis of this study. John O'Hare, Michael Klausner, and Matthew Gelfand provided research assistance. David Padgett and Christine de Fontenay wrote the computer program to glean data from the American Hospital Association's hospital survey tapes. Charlotte Kaiser typed the manuscript. Evelyn Fisher, with the help of Amy Raths, verified its factual content. Florence Robinson prepared the index.

The study was financed by a grant from the National Science Foundation. The views expressed here are the author's alone and should not be ascribed to the officers, trustees, or other staff members of the Brookings Institution, to the National Science Foundation, or to any of those who were consulted or who commented on the manuscript.

BRUCE K. MAC LAURY
President

February 1979
Washington, D.C.

Contents

Figures

chapter one Introduction

At the time it must have seemed as though the decade of the sixties, a decade of optimism about the perfectibility of the human race, would see the conquest of disease by medical science. Not so many years earlier, the miracle drugs—sulfa, penicillin, and other antibiotics—had been discovered. In the 1950s, the iron lung, itself a recently developed life-saving technology, was made obsolete by the vaccine for polio. Through the 1950s and the 1960s, a host of new medical treatments appeared, often based on impressively complex machinery—the pacemaker, the artificial kidney, open-heart surgery, coronary care units, kidney and heart transplants. Each new discovery was accompanied by excitement, publicity, and renewed hope. While the 1970s came and disease was not yet conquered, there was still a sense of rapid progress: new funds were committed to cancer research in the belief that important advances were within reach and only money was needed to achieve them, and the first artificial hearts were implanted in human beings.

During the same years that these technologies were being introduced the amount of money the nation spent on medical care was rising, faster than the gross national product, and with increased speed after the mid-1960s. The statistic that has probably drawn the most attention is the cost of a day in the hospital, which was about $14 in 1950 and had risen to $151 by 1976.[1] Total national expenditures for all types of medical care grew from $12 billion in 1950, to $39 billion in 1965, and $139 billion in 1976 (data are for fiscal years). When these amounts are expressed as a proportion of GNP, it is clear that medical care has been claiming a growing share of the country's real resources: this share was 4.5 percent

1. This is the cost per patient day after subtracting the costs of outpatient visits. Without this adjustment, the numbers are $16 and $173, respectively. The data necessary to make the adjustment are not available for years before 1965, so the $14 estimate for 1950 was derived using the same proportional adjustment as for 1965.

in 1950, 5.9 percent of a considerably larger GNP in 1965, and 8.6 percent—almost double the figure for 1950—in 1976.[2]

The steady growth of costs has come to be perceived as a serious problem: costs are "too high" and growing "too fast." The federal medical care programs passed in the 1960s, of which Medicare and Medicaid are the largest, have found themselves spending far more than originally forecast and putting demands on the budget that leave no room for new programs. Health insurance provided by employers as a fringe benefit to their employees has become so expensive that it is a major issue in collective bargaining.

When one looks around for explanations for the growth in costs, new technologies stand out as an obvious possibility. Many of them are indeed very expensive. The cost of an open-heart procedure is estimated at between $10,000 and $15,000. Kidney dialysis for a year costs $7,000 or more if it is done at home and between $15,000 and $25,000 if it is done in an outpatient clinic, as it is for most dialysis patients. The cost of a day in a coronary care unit is several times the cost of a day in an ordinary hospital bed.

But new technologies are only some of the things we spend our money on, not the reason we spend it—a symptom, not a cause. The real reason for the rising costs is much more general and has to do with the growth of private health insurance and public programs like Medicare and Medicaid, referred to collectively as third party payers.

The growth of third party payment has been most extensive for hospital care—the most costly and unpredictable kind of medical care. In 1950, between 40 and 50 percent of hospital costs were paid through third party payers, with the rest paid directly by the patient. In the years that followed, more people bought private insurance or received it as a fringe benefit of employment. Medicare and Medicaid were passed in 1965 to help the aged and the poor, two groups whose medical expenses were so high or whose incomes so low—sometimes both—that they found it difficult to buy insurance. By the mid-1970s, 90 percent of all hospital costs were paid through third party payers and only 10 percent directly by patients.

Third party payment arises out of the philosophy that no one should have to forgo medical care that might save his life or preserve his health because he cannot afford to pay. As a means for putting this philosophy

2. Robert M. Gibson and Marjorie Smith Mueller, "National Health Expenditure Highlights, Fiscal Year 1976," Research and Statistics Note 27 (Social Security Administration, December 22, 1976), p. 2.

into practice, it has been thoroughly successful. Most people today do not have to worry about whether they can afford hospital care when they need it.

The opposite side of the coin is that, because they pay little or nothing directly for hospital care, and because their own decisions about care have no perceptible effect on the insurance premiums and taxes they pay, people draw on resources as though they cost nothing. Translated into the everyday terms of patients and doctors, third party payment says "Use whatever might be beneficial and do not concern yourselves with how great the costs may be or how small the benefits." This is not a distortion of the original philosophy. It is precisely what was intended, but the consequences have never been fully appreciated. In particular, it has never been appreciated that when benefits do not have to be weighed against costs—when the only criterion is that there be *some* benefit—the number of good things that can be done in medical care is, for all practical purposes, unlimited.

Freed of economic restraints by third party payment, the medical sector in general—and hospitals in particular, since third party payment is most extensive for hospital care—has pulled in new resources almost as fast as it can separate them from other areas of the economy, in order to provide all the care that might be of some benefit. The resulting flow of resources has been the primary component in rising expenditures. Wages and prices higher than those elsewhere in the economy—which are necessary in some degree to attract the new resources into the sector—have been only minor contributors.[3]

A few statistics can illustrate how important the flow of resources has been. About half of each year's increase in cost per hospital day, which has exceeded 12 percent on average since 1965, has been due to the rising level of resources used per day. In consequence, this level approximately *doubled* between 1965 and 1978. As a more concrete example of the growth in resources, the number of people employed in short-stay hospitals—those necessary to staff new beds as well as those attributable to higher levels of staff per bed—grew 79 percent between 1965 and 1976, from 1.4 million to 2.5 million. The number of employees per bed increased 38 percent over the same period, from 1.9 to 2.6.

The age-old economic problem—unlimited wants, limited means—has thus not been done away with by third party payment, but only recast

3. Martin Feldstein and Amy Taylor, *The Rapid Rise of Hospital Costs* (Executive Office of the President, Council on Wage and Price Stability, January 1977).

in more aggregate terms. There is no end to the good things that can be done, or attempted, in medical care; even with all that is being spent, there are still many people who could benefit from more or better care than they are now getting. Because of third party payment patients and their doctors can pursue the best care largely without economic constraint. But society is then faced with the result of these individual decisions: medical care is claiming a growing share of its limited resources, and at the aggregate level it is more difficult to maintain the fiction encouraged at the individual level, that resources are unlimited. At the aggregate level it is more obvious that the resources used for medical care are resources taken from some other purpose.

As we consider whether to modify the philosophy that no one should have to forgo medical care because of its cost, and if so how to modify it, we have to begin to ask a new set of questions. What are we getting in return for the resources committed to medical care? Who benefits and how much? How do we value these benefits as compared to other ways we might use the resources? How might we go about limiting the resources available for medical care, if we decide to do so?

This study is about the new technologies that have been introduced in hospitals over the last twenty-five years. The purpose of the study is not to single them out as the "cause" of the cost problem but to ask some of the questions and begin to supply some of the answers that are necessary if the flow of resources into medical care is not to be allowed to continue unrestrained, and to ask these questions about things which, perhaps more than any others, we had hoped could be left untouched—the "miracles" of modern medicine.

The approach combines case study and statistical methods. A number of specific technologies are considered from both points of view. The case study of each technology looks at its purpose and use, its history, the kinds and amounts of resources it employs and their cost, and its benefits for patients. The case studies repeatedly demonstrate the truth of the general description of the cost problem just given: in the presence of extensive third party payment, investment in a technology will continue until the benefit from any further investment is zero.

The explanation itself is not new,[4] but the case studies offer fresh evi-

4. See, in particular, the works of Martin S. Feldstein, for example, "Hospital Cost Inflation: A Study of Nonprofit Price Dynamics," *American Economic Review,* vol. 61 (December 1971), pp. 853–72; and "The High Cost of Hospitals— And What to Do About It," *Public Interest,* no. 48 (Summer 1977), pp. 40–54.

dence for it, and evidence of a sort that helps bring out the nature of the choices that face us if we do decide to limit the growth of medical care costs.

The statistical analysis investigates the distribution of the technology among hospitals, or when the data permit, the speed with which it was adopted, and tries to explain what factors account for that distribution and that speed. It is unable to add much to our understanding of third party payment because of the inadequacies of the data on this point. But it produces evidence about a number of other important factors—including medical education, research, and perhaps of greatest interest, past attempts by federal and state governments to influence the adoption of new technologies by hospitals.

The work is organized into six chapters. The next chapter, chapter 2, steps aside from the main stream of the book to give the background for the statistical analyses. It describes the metropolitan hospitals on which the analyses are based. Data on the hospitals themselves from the surveys of the American Hospital Association (AHA), and data on the metropolitan areas and the states in which they are located are presented and discussed. Some readers may prefer to skip this chapter at first and refer back to it only as questions about the data occur to them.

The three chapters that follow consider particular technologies, or groups of technologies, beginning in each case with the case study of the technology and finishing with the statistical work. Chapter 3 is devoted to the major forms of intensive care—the postoperative recovery room, the mixed intensive care unit, and the coronary care unit. Although it is less often in the headlines than more exotic technologies such as organ transplants, intensive care is a very important and very expensive technology in modern hospital care. The chapter includes a separate section about the benefits of intensive care, both because the subject is important in its own right and because it has something to say about a crucial aspect of making decisions about any medical technology—evaluating its benefits for the patient.

Chapter 4 considers the speed with which three quite different but now quite common technologies—respiratory therapy, diagnostic radioisotopes, and the electroencephalograph—were adopted during the 1960s and the first half of the 1970s. Chapter 5 looks at the current distribution of three rather more unusual technologies—open-heart surgery, cobalt therapy, and renal dialysis (kidney dialysis)—which are still found primarily in large hospitals. Because they are less common, the most important years of their diffusion were not picked up by the AHA surveys and it is not possible to analyze the speed of this process.

The United States is not alone in facing the dilemma posed by new medical technologies. Chapter 6 looks at the policies of four countries— the United States, Sweden, Great Britain, and France—for dealing, directly or indirectly, with decisions about medical technologies. It measures these policies against a framework that describes the stages of thought as nations come to grips with the nature of the problem. Most countries, and three of the four considered at length in the chapter, have yet to relinquish the hope that containing costs is consistent with providing everything that might be beneficial to everyone who might benefit from it. Only Great Britain has abandoned that view and adopted instead the objective of limiting resources but making the limited resources equally available.

The final chapter, chapter 7, summarizes and discusses the conclusions of the study.

chapter two Hospitals and Hospital Markets

The decisions that the administration and medical staff of a hospital make about particular technologies depend on what they see as the most important purposes of the institution and on the characteristics of its environment that shape those purposes or that make them more or less difficult to pursue. All hospitals have as their primary function the treatment of sick people, and for many this is their only function. How they carry it out will be influenced by the types of people they see most often and the types they would like to see—patterns that reflect the philosophies and special training of the doctors affiliated with them. A minority of hospitals, usually large ones, combine patient care with the education of students in the health professions—doctors, nurses, dentists, technicians of various sorts—and some commit themselves to research programs of varying degrees of intensity and sophistication. In all of these pursuits, they are constrained by external forces, particularly the ease or difficulty of getting money to finance their plans and the types of regulation imposed by the governments with jurisdiction over them.

In the briefest possible outline, this is the framework that underlies the statistical analyses of chapters 3, 4, and 5. This chapter fills in the details of the outline by describing the features of hospitals and their environments that seem likely to affect the adoption of new technologies. In the course of the discussion, most of the data used to represent these characteristics in the subsequent analyses are presented, and the strengths and weaknesses of the data as proxies for the desired characteristics are explained.

Selection of Hospitals and Definition of Markets

There are more than 6,000 short-term, acute-care, hospitals—hospitals that provide general medical care—in the United States, and they decide the fate of new technologies intended for use in hospitals.[1] Some of these, fewer than 400 in 1976, are federal hospitals and are open only to special groups of people—members of the armed services and their families and certain groups of veterans, for example. The rest, 5,956 in 1976, with 961,000 beds in all, are nonfederal hospitals open to the general public. These are what the American Hospital Association calls community hospitals, and the term will be used in this study as well.

There are three general sorts of ownership-management arrangements among community hospitals. The majority—57 percent in 1976—are nonprofit institutions, and these account for an even larger share of the beds in community hospitals, about 70 percent in 1976. Hospitals run by state, county, or city governments make up another 31 percent of the hospitals and supply 22 percent of the beds. Hospitals operated for profit account for the remaining 13 percent of community hospitals and 8 percent of the beds.

Under the definition of short term adopted by the AHA, the average stay in community hospitals is less than thirty days. The overwhelming majority of these hospitals are general service institutions, meaning that they accept people of any age with virtually any condition. A handful are more specialized—children's hospitals, for example, obstetrical hospitals, or ear, nose, and throat hospitals.

With the exception of a relatively few major medical centers that draw patients from all over, hospitals operate in local markets delimited by the practice boundaries of physicians and the distances patients must travel. Since many of the influences that affect decisions about technologies are peculiar to these market areas, the data should refer to them. But it is impossible to determine the exact market boundaries for each hospital in a study that covers as many hospitals as this one does. Luckily a reasonable approximation to local hospital markets is available for metropolitan areas, in the form of the standard metropolitan statistical areas defined by the federal government as a common standard for the presentation of data collected by government agencies.

Standard metropolitan statistical areas (SMSAs) are collections of

---

1. In 1976 there were 746 hospitals other than short-term hospitals: 528 were nonfederal psychiatric hospitals, 197 were nonfederal hospitals specializing in the long-term care of the chronically ill, and 21 were nonfederal hospitals for tuberculosis and other respiratory diseases. In addition, a few of the 380 federal hospitals should probably be classified as other than short term, but the data do not permit them to be separated from the total.

contiguous urban counties.[2] A county is included in an SMSA when a certain fraction of its citizens work elsewhere in the SMSA, and/or a certain fraction of its labor force is drawn from other parts of the SMSA. This implies established patterns of travel that can reasonably be expected to carry over into hospital use and hospital employment. In all, about three-quarters of the U.S. population lives in SMSAs. Metropolitan hospitals account for almost precisely half of all community hospitals; but because they are much larger than rural hospitals, on average, their share of beds in community hospitals—about three-quarters—is quite in keeping with the size of the population they serve.

To begin then, the hospitals selected for analysis were limited to those located in SMSAs. The definitions of SMSAs are revised from time to time to reflect the constant growth and change of cities, but for the purposes of this study the definitions established in 1975 were used throughout the collection of data and the selection of hospitals.[3] A total of 256 SMSAs are used in this study.

The information about the individual hospitals in these SMSAs came from the annual surveys of the American Hospital Association (AHA) for the years 1961 through 1975. The AHA surveys all the hospitals in the country and the response is quite good—generally over 90 percent for

2. The first part of the detailed definition of an SMSA reads: "Each standard metropolitan statistical area must include at least: (a) One city with 50,000 or more inhabitants, or (b) A city with at least 25,000 inhabitants, which, together with those contiguous places . . . having population densities of at least 1,000 persons per square mile, has a combined population of 50,000 and constitutes for general economic and social purposes a single community, provided that the county or counties in which the city and contiguous places are located has a total population of at least 75,000." The second and third parts of the definition set out the criteria used to determine whether contiguous counties should be considered to form a single community. Office of Management and Budget, *Standard Metropolitan Statistical Areas, 1975,* rev. ed. (Government Printing Office, 1976), pp. 1–2.

3. Three adjustments were made in these definitions. First, the two SMSAs in Alaska and Hawaii were omitted because not all of the data sources used for the study included them. Second, two Virginia SMSAs (Petersburg-Colonial Heights-Hopewell and Richmond) were combined because the complications introduced by the existence of independent cities within counties in Virginia made it impossible to separate some of the data for these SMSAs into mutually exclusive sets. Third, for New England, SMSAs are defined in terms of townships rather than counties. Since data for many of the characteristics of interest were available only by county, the alternative metropolitan areas defined for New England by the federal government—called New England county metropolitan areas—were used instead. The term standard metropolitan statistical area, or SMSA, is used to refer to all of the resulting 256 metropolitan areas. (See ibid. for definitions.)

all hospitals (in 1975, it was 92 percent) and higher for hospitals with 100 or more beds (in 1975, the response rate was better than 95 percent for these hospitals). The questionnaire asks for information about such things as costs, employment, and admissions during the year, and, of greatest importance, about the facilities and services available in the hospital—intensive care units, cobalt therapy, renal dialysis, and the like.

In 1975, a total of 2,772 community hospitals were located in an SMSA and filled in the AHA's questionnaire. These hospitals, and the SMSAs in which they were located, were the basis for the analyses of the distribution of technologies across hospitals in 1975, analyses that attempt to determine what characteristics of the hospital and its market are associated with having, or not having, a particular technology (chapters 3 and 5).[4] A second set of hospitals, 2,770 in all, was made up of those community hospitals in SMSAs that responded to the survey in at least ten of the fifteen years from 1961 through 1975.[5] The hospitals that adopted certain technologies during those years were then selected from this second set and used to analyze the speed of adoption. Chapters 3 and 4, which describe these analyses, give the number of hospitals available in each case.

The 2,772 hospitals selected from the 1975 survey were 93 percent of all metropolitan hospitals in that year, and, as table 2-1 shows, 47 percent of all community hospitals. They included the overwhelming majority of large hospitals—over 90 percent of those with 300 or more beds. Most of them were general service hospitals; only 5.4 percent classified themselves as a more specialized type of institution. About 69 percent were nonprofit, 16 percent were run by state, county, or city governments, and 15 percent were operated for profit. As the national statistics mentioned earlier suggest, the ownership-management of rural hospitals is quite different, with local government institutions much more important and nonprofit ones much less so.

The market area characteristics constitute the bulk of the potential explanatory factors, and the tables that accompany the discussion in the

4. As it turned out, none of the hospitals in one of the 256 SMSAs (Santa Cruz, California) completed the questionnaire in 1975, so they and their SMSA do not contribute to the analyses based on that year. The tables in this chapter, however, show all 256 SMSAs because the hospitals in Santa Cruz did respond to earlier surveys and may therefore be present in some of the analyses that cover the period 1961–75.

5. The time series extends back only to 1961 because the surveys for earlier years have not been recorded on computer tape by the AHA.

Table 2-1. Distribution of Community Hospitals[a] in the United States and
Those Used in the Study, by Size, 1975

Beds in hospital	Number of hospitals		Study hospitals as percent of total
	Used in study	Total in United States	
1–49	260	1,454	17.9
50–99	450	1,481	30.4
100–199	727	1,363	53.3
200–299	505	678	74.5
300–399	334	378	88.4
400–499	217	230	94.3
500 and over	279	291	95.9
All hospitals	2,772	5,875	47.2

Sources: Total hospitals, *Hospital Statistics, 1976 Edition: Data from American Hospital Association 1975 Annual Survey;* study hospitals, tabulated from American Hospital Association's 1975 survey of hospitals.

a. Community hospitals are nonfederal short-term hospitals. The numbers shown exclude hospital units of institutions.

rest of the chapter present the distributions of these characteristics for the 256 SMSAs. This is the best way to show the amount of variation in the data since the values are, of course, the same for all hospitals in the same SMSA. But the reader will want to know as well how the 2,772 hospitals, which are the basis for the regressions, were distributed for each characteristic. These distributions are given in appendix A, in detail that matches the intervals used in the analysis but in less detail than shown in this chapter.

With a few exceptions, the emphasis in the discussion is on the differences between areas rather than on changes over time. In most cases, interarea differences change slowly, and thus one or at most two years of data are sufficient to represent a longer time period (and in several cases the data are sums or averages over several years). Further, for some of the technologies, the fact that the hospital has them is known, but the year in which they were introduced is not, because the AHA first asked about them some time after their adoption. For these technologies, changes over time in the explanatory variables could not be related accurately to the adoption of the technology in any event.

For both these reasons it was not considered important to use a common year for all the data, and the choice of year was based on considerations of availability and quality peculiar to the individual items. In general, however, the years cluster in the late 1960s. These years are about midway through the fifteen-year period covered by the surveys (1961–75).

Thus they are as good a choice as many others for the analysis based on the 1975 hospital survey and are particularly appropriate for the analysis of the diffusion over time of the technologies for which such an analysis is possible.

The discussion of the data is organized along the lines outlined earlier. First, the possible purposes and functions of a hospital—the care of patients and the intervening influence of the doctors who care for them, education, and research—are considered, then the competitive structure of the hospital market, followed by the sources of financing for hospital investment, and finally the various forms of intervention and regulation attempted by governments.

The Hospital's Objectives

Economists generally assume that the primary objective of most businesses is to make money for their owners—in more formal terms, to maximize profits. This has the advantage for statistical research that it is easy to represent the profitability of a technology, or any other action, in numeric terms and then measure its effect on the firm's subsequent behavior. For example, in his study of the diffusion of new technologies in railroading, steel, coal mining, and brewing, Mansfield was able to measure the profits expected from each innovation and show that the higher they were, the more quickly the technology was adopted.[6]

Because so many hospitals are legally designated nonprofit institutions and have no owners or shareholders to receive profits, economists and the public, with a few exceptions, have concluded that they do not try to maximize profits. The literature on what their goals might be instead is vague. Beyond reiterating that hospitals probably do not aim for profits, it suggests only that their objectives are numerous and probably combine elements of the quantity of care—the number of days of care is usually mentioned—with aspects of its quality.[7] What aspects of quality might be important, or how they might be measured, are left, for all practical purposes, to the reader's imagination.

6. Edwin Mansfield, *Industrial Research and Technological Innovation: An Econometric Analysis* (Norton, 1968), chap. 7.

7. Karen Davis, "Economic Theories of Behavior in Nonprofit, Private Hospitals," *Economic and Business Bulletin,* vol. 24 (Winter 1972), pp. 1–13 (Brookings Reprint 239).

The situation being what it is, with no professional consensus to turn to, this study takes an empirical and exploratory approach to the matter of hospital objectives. As a starting point it seems reasonable to assert that, whatever a hospital's objectives are, they are closely related to the three possible functions listed earlier—the care of patients, teaching, and research—and that for most hospitals the care of patients is first among these. Thus the statistical work is based on data that measure what seem on the basis of common sense to be reasonable representatives of these functions.

To begin, a hospital's decisions will certainly be influenced by the scale of its operations. The number of beds in the hospital is used in the statistical analysis as a proxy for this scale, which is reflected in the number of patients, the number of doctors affiliated with the hospital, the number of residents in training, and so on. The rest of the data representing the hospital's objectives are then expressed *relative to* the number of beds, on the supposition that a hospital will behave differently from other hospitals operating on the same scale only if, for example, the characteristics of its patients or the relative size of its residency programs differ from the average for those hospitals.

The Care of Patients

Some technologies are specific to the diagnosis or treatment of certain diseases, and a hospital may be influenced in its decision to adopt one of them by the incidence of the disease in its community. For example, heart disease and cancer, which are, respectively, the first- and second-ranked causes of death in the United States, make up a substantial portion of hospital admissions, and several of the technologies considered in this study—especially intensive care, open-heart surgery, and cobalt therapy —are directed at their treatment.

Table 2-2 presents data on deaths from cancer and heart disease among the residents of each SMSA, per 1,000 beds in short-term hospitals in the SMSA,[8] and, more conventionally, per 100,000 people in the SMSA.[9] The range in both measures is wide, with the highest rates five to ten times

8. Since the deaths include those of people treated in federal hospitals, the number of beds includes federal as well as nonfederal short-term hospitals.

9. These rates have not been adjusted for age and sex (as is usually done in the publications of the National Institutes of Health, which supplied the data) because it is assumed that what is important to the hospital is the actual number of cases it might attract, not some adjusted number.

Table 2-2. Distributions of Standard Metropolitan Statistical Areas by Deaths from Cancer and Heart Disease

	Number of SMSAs by cause of death	
Annual deaths[a]	Cancer	Heart disease
Per 1,000 short-term hospital beds[b]		
50–99	6	1
100–199	62	6
200–299	96	18
300–399	65	48
400–499	22	51
500–599	5	54
600–699	...	39
700 and over	...	39
Total	256	256
Per 100,000 population		
50–99	29	1
100–149	134	27
150–199	85	54
200–249	8	91
250–299	...	61
300 and over	...	22
Total	256	256

Sources: Data on deaths from cancer are from Thomas J. Mason and Frank W. McKay, *U.S. Cancer Mortality by County: 1950–1969*, National Institutes of Health, DHEW (NIH) 74-615 (Government Printing Office, 1974); data on deaths from heart disease were supplied by the National Heart, Lung, and Blood Institute; data on beds are from the AHA's 1969 survey of hospitals.

a. The original data were the total numbers of deaths for 1950–69 in the case of cancer and for 1968–71 in the case of heart disease. They have been adjusted to show annual averages. Deaths from heart disease are for persons thirty-five to seventy-four years old.

b. In federal and nonfederal hospitals, 1969.

larger than the lowest. It is wider for the rates per 1,000 hospital beds, where relatively large numbers of deaths may combine with relatively small numbers of beds—and vice versa—to produce the extreme values, than for the rates per 100,000 people. Nonetheless, many of the SMSAs in which deaths are high relative to hospital capacity are those one would predict from the per capita rates. For example, the eight SMSAs with more than 900 deaths from heart disease per 1,000 hospital beds include three in Florida—Tampa-St. Petersburg, Fort Lauderdale, and Fort Myers.

The number of people who die from a disease is not, of course, the same as the number who have it. But data on incidence are not available, and, for two such serious diseases, it seems reasonable to believe that death rates are a good proxy for incidence—or at least for those especially serious cases that, sooner or later, end up in the hospital. This is particularly true for cancer: unlike heart disease, cancer does not kill people so quickly that they have no chance to get to a hospital, and national averages show that the number of deaths every year is more than one-third the number of people being treated for cancer.[10]

The death rates for heart disease and cancer are averages across each SMSA and are not specific to particular hospitals in it. While in some cases, SMSA data are used because no information is available for hospitals, in this case they are to be preferred. The aim is to measure the number of patients the hospital thought it might be able to attract if it adopted the technology, not the number it did attract after it adopted the technology. Looking at the data in table 2-2 again, this time from the point of view of the individual hospital, one can see that the variation in, for example, cancer deaths suggests that a 200-bed hospital in an SMSA in the lowest interval (50 through 99 deaths per 1,000 beds) might admit no more than ten or twenty patients dying of cancer during a year, while a hospital of the same size in one of the SMSAs at the other end of the distribution (500 through 599 deaths per 1,000 beds) might admit 100 or more. The total number of cases treated during a year would average about three times the number of deaths.

Death rates from respiratory diseases and motor vehicle accidents (not shown in this chapter) are used in the analysis of certain technologies. But for some technologies there are no data on the diseases the technology is designed to treat. For these, the number of people per short-term hospital bed in the SMSA (table 2-3) is used as a rough proxy for potential patients. Where the number of people per bed is higher, there may be more pressure on the available beds, with the result that a higher proportion of patients admitted to the hospital may have the serious conditions for which sophisticated technologies are used.

The ratio extends from a low of 53 people per bed in Rochester, Minnesota (the next observations are over 90) to values approximately ten times higher in Fort Collins, Colorado (508) and Bryan-College Station, Texas (547). In terms of the more familiar ratio of beds to population, the range runs down from nearly nineteen beds per 1,000 population in

10. The number of deaths is about 150 per 100,000 persons per year, compared to 430 cases under treatment per 100,000. See Ned B. Hornback, L. E. Cloe, and David J. Edwards, "Report of Radiation Therapy and Therapeutic Radioisotope Facilities and Personnel in Indiana: A Model for Projecting Need in 1980," *Journal of the Indiana State Medical Association,* vol. 69 (July 1976), pp. 508–09.

Table 2-3. Distribution of Standard Metropolitan Statistical Areas by Population per Hospital Bed, 1969–70

Population per short-term hospital bed[a]	Number of SMSAs
50–99	4
100–149	20
150–199	64
200–249	72
250–299	59
300–349	23
350–399	6
400–449	4
450–499	2
500–549	2
Total	256

Sources: Population figures are census data from a tape provided by Department of Health, Education, and Welfare; number of beds, AHA's 1969 survey of hospitals.

a. 1970 resident population divided by beds in all short-term hospitals, federal and nonfederal, in 1969.

Rochester to slightly fewer than two per 1,000 in Bryan-College Station. (The national average in 1970 was just under five short-term beds per 1,000.) The use of persons per bed as a proxy for the incidence of disease is lent credibility by the fact that it is highly correlated with cancer and heart disease deaths per 1,000 beds (0.60 and 0.68, respectively).

The composition of an SMSA's population in terms of age, sex, and race can also help to represent differences in the incidence of diseases for which direct measures are not available. And even when good proxies for incidence are available, as in the cases of heart disease and cancer, these attributes can represent the personal characteristics of sick people that reflect differences in the kind of care they need. For example, if elderly people take longer to recuperate, a hospital with a high proportion of elderly patients will have, at any one time, relatively fewer patients who require intensive or sophisticated services.

Table 2-4 shows the distributions of the 256 SMSAs for the proportions of their populations that are sixty-five years old or older, female, and white. In most SMSAs the proportion sixty-five years or older falls between 5 and 10 percent (the national proportion in 1970 was 9.8 percent), but it is greater than 10 percent in a sizable number, and greater than 15 percent in eight. Many of the SMSAs with extreme values are, of course, in Florida, including all three in which more than 20 percent of the population is sixty-five years or older. The percent female is almost entirely concentrated in the interval 50 through 54 percent; with so little variation among SMSAs it is not surprising that it turned out to have no influence on the adoption of technologies. By contrast, the proportion of the population that is white varies from a low of 59 percent in Pine Bluff, Arkansas, to a high of virtually 100 percent in Dubuque, Iowa.

The link between the characteristics of potential patients and the cases actually admitted to a hospital is usually indirect. Physicians act as intermediaries, translating the patient's demand for medical care into a demand for the services of particular hospitals, and they have their own reasons for wanting new and advanced technologies. Some of these reasons may correspond closely to the characteristics of the patients. Some may not: the scope that a well-equipped hospital gives them in their practice, the prestige and sense of security attached to working in a hospital

Table 2-4. Distributions of Standard Metropolitan Statistical Areas by Age, Sex, and Race, 1970

	Number of SMSAs by patient characteristic		
Percent	*Sixty-five years or older*	*Female*	*White*
1–4	4	...	...
5–9	168	...	...
10–14	76	...	...
15–19	5	...	...
20–24	2	...	...
25–29	1	...	...
30–34	...	...	...
35–39	...	...	...
40–44	...	3	...
45–49	...	25	...
50–54	...	228	...
55–59	...	...	1
60–64	...	...	3
65–69	...	...	7
70–74	...	...	17
75–79	...	...	14
80–84	...	...	25
85–89	...	...	37
90–94	...	...	67
95–100	...	...	85
Total	256	256	256

Source: Percentages are derived from census data from a tape provided by the Department of Health, Education, and Welfare.

that has all the latest facilities, and the additional income this allows them to earn. Whatever the precise reasons, they mean that the adoption of technologies by hospitals is likely to be influenced by the numbers and kinds of physicians on its staff at the time the decisions are being made.

In this case, data for the individual hospital would probably be best, as long as the data represented the staff of the hospital at the time the technology was being considered and not at some later date. (The information should represent the situation that influenced the hospital in its decision, not the situation that resulted from it.) Data are available to meet the second requirement—that they should precede the year of the dependent variable by a wide margin—but not the first. It was only possible to get data for SMSAs, not individual hospitals.

The statistics used are for 1968, seven years earlier than the information from the 1975 survey and about midway through the years covered by all fifteen surveys. An earlier year might have been still better, as some technologies—like cobalt therapy—were being adopted well before 1968; but the American Medical Association (AMA) changed its method of classifying physicians in the middle 1960s and this consideration lost out to a preference for data based on the new system. Fortunately, the numbers and specialty distribution of physicians change fairly slowly—this was particularly true until the 1970s, when federal programs to increase the number of physicians began to show results—so that the data for 1968 are probably not much different from those for some years earlier.[11]

Only nonfederal physicians defined by the AMA as engaged in patient care in office-based practice were counted. These are the physicians whose recommendations bring patients to community hospitals (which, the reader will recall, are nonfederal). The remaining physicians in patient care are hospital-based and the bulk of these are interns and residents (61 percent in 1968). Interns and residents represent an influence on technology of a different sort—they are the major part of a hospital's teaching responsibilities—and in any event, separate data are available to represent them.

Table 2-5 shows the number of physicians per 1,000 short-term hospital beds in 1968. The hypothesis here rests on the fact that physicians are

11. In the case of the specialty distribution, this speculation is supported by the high correlations between the SMSA data for 1963 and 1968, in spite of the intervening change in the classification system. The correlations for the percentages of an SMSA's physicians in each of the four specialty groups are: general practice, 0.92; medical specialties, 0.88; surgical specialties, 0.81; other specialties, 0.73.

Table 2-5. Distribution of Standard Metropolitan Statistical Areas by Physicians per 1,000 Hospital Beds, 1968–69

Physicians per 1,000 short-term hospital beds	Number of SMSAs
100–124	9
125–149	28
150–174	37
175–199	39
200–224	40
225–249	29
250–274	35
275–299	11
300–324	10
325–349	5
350–374	5
375–399	3
400–424	2
425–449	3
Total	256

Sources: Number of nonfederal physicians engaged in patient care as of December 31, 1968 (excluding hospital-based physicians), from American Medical Association, *Distribution of Physicians, Hospitals, and Hospital Beds in the U.S., 1968* (AMA, 1969); beds in nonfederal short-term hospitals in 1969, from AHA's 1969 survey of hospitals.

attracted by, and want more of, the latest in equipment and facilities. Where there are more physicians—hence more wants—relative to bed capacity, hospitals may be under greater pressure to adopt new technologies. This pressure is reinforced by the fact that, where there are more physicians, more patients will be seen and diagnosed as needing some form of hospital care.[12] Not surprisingly, the SMSAs at the low end of the distribution include many in the Plains states, which have fewer doctors and more hospital beds than many other states, while those at the high end include many with university medical centers—San Francisco, New York, New Haven, Ann Arbor, Washington, D.C., and so on.

To some extent, a physician's specialty will determine the particular kinds of facilities he wants. For example, where there are more physicians in the surgical specialties, there may be more pressure for things like open-heart surgery units. The medical specialties are dominated numerically by internists and pediatricians, but they include specialists in cardiology,

12. The number of hospital beds is not necessarily a constraint on the use of hospital facilities since some facilities—radiotherapy and respiratory therapy are examples—serve many outpatients.

Table 2-6. Distributions of Standard Metropolitan Statistical Areas by Percent of Physicians in Four Specialty Groups, 1968[a]

Percent in specialty group	Number of SMSAs by physician specialty			
	General practice	Medical specialties	Surgical specialties	Other specialties
0–4	1	...	...	...
5–9	...	1	...	9
10–14	15	21	...	69
15–19	33	63	1	126
20–24	59	103	2	46
25–29	62	57	54	4
30–34	46	10	101	2
35–39	19	...	72	...
40–44	12	1	22	...
45–54	9	...	4	...
Total	256	256	256	256

Source: AMA, *Distribution of Physicians, Hospitals, and Hospital Beds in the U.S., 1968.*
a. Nonfederal physicians engaged in patient care as of December 31, 1968, excluding hospital-based physicians.

who will want coronary care units, and specialists in pulmonary disease, who will want respiratory therapy departments. Other specialists include those in diagnostic and therapeutic radiology, and several of the facilities considered in this study fall into their jurisdiction. The distribution of physicians by specialty serves as an approximation to these preferences— a rather rough one since the four specialty groups reported by the AMA are fairly broad.

The proportions of physicians in each of the four groups vary widely across SMSAs (table 2-6). The proportion in general practice covers the widest range—from Rochester, Minnesota, at the extreme low end, with only 2.8 percent of its physicians in general practice, to York and Lancaster, Pennsylvania, each with more than 50 percent. The variation in the other three groups, while less, is still substantial. Surgeons account for the largest share of doctors, with 101 SMSAs having 30 to 34 percent of their physicians in these specialties. The SMSAs at the extremes in numbers of surgeons have in common that they are small (for example, Anderson, Indiana, with 20 percent, and Elmira, New York, with 48 percent) suggesting that, in cities with relatively small numbers of physicians, accidents of history may result in a skewed specialty distribution. SMSAs with proportionately few physicians in the medical specialties also tend to be small, but those with proportionately many are a mixture, including some large SMSAs, and that inveterate extremist, Rochester, Minnesota, with 44 percent.[13]

Teaching and Research

There were 114 medical schools in the United States in 1975, virtually all of them in metropolitan areas. Several SMSAs had more than one school—New York City claimed seven—while close to three-quarters had none. The hospitals affiliated with these schools are, by virtue of the connection, involved in varying degrees in the education of undergraduate medical students, in residency training, and in the clinical aspects of medical research.

The AHA survey provides information about two important aspects of each hospital's involvement in education: its affiliation with a medical school and the number of residents on its staff. Of the 2,772 nonfederal metropolitan hospitals taken from the 1975 survey, 629 reported that they were affiliated with a medical school. Medical students ordinarily spend most of the last two of their four undergraduate years in these hospitals getting the clinical part of their education. This education takes the form of ward rounds, "a sort of strolling seminar" led by one of the practicing physicians with admitting privileges at the hospital, and the students practice going through the diagnostic routines with some of the patients seen on the rounds. In the course of the two years, each student experiences all of the major specialties in the hospital—internal medicine, surgery, pediatrics, obstetrics-gynecology, and psychiatry.[14]

Although residency training is concentrated in hospitals affiliated with medical schools, it is not limited to these. Over 30 percent of the study hospitals (876) reported they employed residents in 1975.[15] During the period of residency (the AMA has dropped the term "internship" in recognition of the fact that virtually no one stops with the legal minimum of one year of postgraduate clinical work any more), physicians get the further clinical training they need to qualify for practice in their specialties. It is possible to do this in as few as two years, but three or four years is standard, and more is quite common, the exact number depending in

13. Rochester is the home of the Mayo Clinic.
14. Robert Lee, "Quality, Location, and Information in Medical Residency Selection" (Ph.D. dissertation, Johns Hopkins University, 1979).
15. This may understate the number of hospitals, as some with programs may not have filled out this part of the questionnaire.

large part on the specialty. At any one time, a hospital will have residents at several different stages of training on its staff.

The numbers of residents reported by hospitals thus differ considerably, reflecting not only the size of the programs but the number and complexity of the specialties in which training is offered. And it seems likely that the more complex the training, the more incentive hospitals have to adopt technologies that complement that training. Of the 876 hospitals reporting residents, 506 had fewer than ten residents per 100 beds in the hospital, 205 had between ten and twenty residents per bed, and 165 had twenty or more.

Medical schools are centers of biomedical research and receive the bulk of the federal funds for that purpose, which further influences the hospitals affiliated with them. Research has become very important since World War II. National expenditures grew from $161 million in 1950 to $4.6 billion in 1975, led by the budget of the National Institutes of Health, the arm of the Department of Health, Education, and Welfare to and through which Congress has funneled increasing amounts of research money. In 1975 the NIH spent $1.7 billion, over half in the form of grants.[16]

About 80 percent of these grant funds are awarded to universities (one-third) and medical schools (two-thirds). Only about 10 percent go directly to hospitals. But because the grants that go to schools affect the climate in which affiliated hospitals operate, and because the distinctions among grants in terms of the institution that formally receives them can be fairly arbitrary (for example, a grant to a component of a university medical center may be formally awarded to the center, or even the university) data were collected on grants to all institutions as well as grants to hospitals. Some of the effect of research is, of course, captured by the simple fact of affiliation with a medical school. The data on grant funds, like the data on residents, offer the chance to distinguish among hospitals in terms of the intensity of their commitment to research.

Unfortunately, the data are available only for SMSAs, not for individual hospitals. Table 2-7 shows the distributions of SMSAs by the

16. Industry contributed more than $1 billion of the $4.6 billion and the rest came from other government agencies and from private nonprofit institutions such as foundations. The data are from Department of Health, Education, and Welfare, National Institutes of Health, *Basic Data Relating to the National Institutes of Health, 1976* (NIH, February 1976); ibid., *1973;* and sources at the National Institutes of Health.

Table 2-7. Distributions of Standard Metropolitan Statistical Areas by National Institutes of Health Research Grant Dollars per Hospital Bed, 1962–75

	Number of SMSAs by type of grant	
Grant dollars[a]	All grants	Grants awarded to hospitals
0	61	153
1–9	6	14
10–49	23	23
50–99	13	12
100–499	40	26
500–999	16	10
1,000–4,999	25	16
5,000–9,999	14	...
10,000–19,999	30	2
20,000–49,999	20	...
50,000 and over	8	...
Total	256	256

Sources: Data on research grants (regular grants; centers, resources, and other grants; and general research support grants), summed over fiscal years 1962–75, supplied by the National Institutes of Health; (grants awarded by institutes no longer part of NIH in 1976 are excluded); number of beds from AHA's 1971 survey of hospitals.

a. In federal and nonfederal short-term hospitals, 1971.

amounts of National Institutes of Health grant dollars awarded over the period 1962–75 relative to the number of short-term hospital beds in the SMSA. Since federal hospitals can receive these grants too, they are included in the denominator. The summing of grants over fourteen years helps insure that the ratios represent the established position of an SMSA, not the isolated success or failure of a single year's grantsmanship.

As the first column of the table shows, the distribution of all grants is uneven. Among those SMSAs that received some funds, forty-two got less than $100 per hospital bed over the fourteen years while eight got more than $50,000. The second column shows the amounts awarded directly to hospitals. The number of SMSAs that received no funds—153—is much larger for this type of award, and the distribution of funds among the remaining SMSAs again covers a wide range.

The Structure of Hospital Markets

Tables 2-8 and 2-9 present two closely related indexes of the competitive structure of metropolitan hospital markets—the number of hospitals in the market and the proportion of beds controlled by the four largest

Table 2-8. Distribution of Standard Metropolitan Statistical Areas by Number of Hospitals, 1975

Hospitals[a]	Number of SMSAs
1	8
2	30
3	32
4	35
5	18
6	20
7	16
8	18
9	11
10–14	27
15–19	9
20 and over	32
Total	256

Source: AHA's 1975 survey of hospitals.
a. All nonfederal short-term hospitals that responded to the 1975 survey.

hospitals (the four-firm concentration ratio). The point was made earlier in the chapter that only nonfederal hospitals are in competition with each other—federal hospitals are limited by law to serving certain specific groups of people who, in turn, have rights to service in those hospitals that they do not have anywhere else. Thus both measures refer only to non-federal hospitals. A few hospitals do not respond to the AHA survey and, for this reason, the number of hospitals may be understated for some SMSAs. But the concentration ratios should be accurate since the response rate is higher for large hospitals than for small ones.

As table 2-8 shows, only eight markets can be classified as monopolies, with a single nonfederal hospital. The rest have two or more hospitals and thus qualify as oligopolies (markets in which there are only a few firms), or some still less concentrated market structure; sixty-eight have ten or more hospitals.

The four-firm concentration ratio measures the extent to which market power in a market with several firms is concentrated in the hands of a few of those firms. The size of the market can be defined in a number of ways —in terms of sales, output, employment, or, as here, in terms of productive capacity. The significance of this ratio in economic thinking lies in the fact that if a few firms account for a large part of the market, this gives them greater power to control the market's production and prices. The

Table 2-9. Distribution of Standard Metropolitan Statistical Areas by Percent of Beds Accounted for by the Four Largest Hospitals, 1975

Percent of beds in four largest hospitals[a]	Number of SMSAs
10–19	7
20–29	5
30–39	16
40–49	8
50–59	11
60–69	20
70–79	26
80–89	26
90–100	67
Market with fewer than four hospitals	70
Total	256

Source: AHA's 1975 survey of hospitals.
a. Nonfederal short-term hospitals.

more concentrated the market, the greater the ability of the few large firms to collaborate successfully.

But the competitive structure of a market depends on factors besides the number and size distribution of firms. It depends as well on the ease with which new firms can enter, the extent to which the firms in a market offer different services, the existence of foreign competition (which for many hospitals may be analogous to the competition offered by regional and national medical centers), and so on. The concentration ratio is only one indicator, and an approximate one at that, of the competitive conditions in each market.

It is partly for this reason that there is disagreement over the value of the four-firm ratio that marks the boundary between markets that are likely to behave in a rivalrous, if not classically competitive, fashion, and those likely to behave more like monopolies. In the context of a discussion of the links between market structure and inflation, Allen reviews several sets of criteria for defining oligopolistic markets, each of which includes a specific value of the four-firm concentration ratio as a major component.[17] One proposal is that a four-firm ratio of 80 percent, maintained

17. Julius W. Allen, "Antitrust Law and Administration: A Survey of Current Issues," *Achieving the Goals of the Employment Act of 1946—Thirtieth Anniversary Review,* vol. 3, no. 2, 94 Cong. 2 sess. (GPO, 1976).

for at least five years, should be considered strong evidence of unreasonable market power. Others set the critical four-firm concentration ratio at 75, 70, and even 50 percent—again usually with the proviso that this ratio should have been maintained for several years.

The concentration ratios in table 2-9 are based on only one year, but they are highly correlated with the ratios for other years and thus offer a reliable clue to the structure of hospital markets.[18] Of the 256 SMSAs, thirty-six meet the most stringent test—a four-firm ratio of less than 50 percent. More than a third, ninety-three in all, qualify as unconcentrated if the dividing line is raised to 80 percent. Because these are the largest and most populous markets, almost three-quarters of the urban population lives in areas where the hospitals, on this measure of market structure, can be considered reasonably competitive.

The significance of the wide variation in market structure for the adoption of technologies remains to be seen. Because of the high level of third party payment for hospital care, it is pointless for hospitals to compete for patients on the basis of price. Studies of regulated industries, in which regulation removes price as a focus for competition, have found that the firms in these industries then compete vigorously on nonprice aspects of service.[19] This suggests that hospitals in less concentrated markets may, other things equal, adopt technologies more frequently and faster than hospitals in oligopolistic and monopolistic markets. But the hypothesis is tentative: the general literature on the effect of market structure on technological diffusion has been unable to come to any accepted conclusions about the links between them.[20]

A more straightforward characteristic of market structure, at least in terms of its expected effect, is the rate of growth of the market. This is represented in the analysis by the growth in the population of the SMSA. A higher rate of growth will encourage hospitals to acquire technologies sooner, or to acquire them when they might not otherwise choose to, in the expectation that even if they are not immediately used to capacity, they soon will be. The distributions of the SMSAs by the growth in population between 1950 and 1970, and between 1960 and 1970, are given in

18. The correlations between the four-firm concentration ratios for 1975, and those for 1970, 1966, and 1961, are 0.98, 0.96, and 0.94, respectively.

19. Roger G. Noll, *Reforming Regulation: An Evaluation of the Ash Council Proposals* (Brookings Institution, 1971).

20. Charles Kennedy and A. P. Thirlwall, "Surveys in Applied Economics: Technical Progress," *Economic Journal,* vol. 82 (March 1972), pp. 11–72.

Table 2-10. Distributions of Standard Metropolitan Statistical Areas by Percent Growth in Population, 1950–70 and 1960–70

	Number of SMSAs by time span	
Percent growth in population	1950–70	1960–70
Negative	7	20
0–9	12	66
10–19	22	80
20–29	31	45
30–39	41	23
40–49	34	8
50–59	30	4
60–69	15	3
70–79	14	1
80–89	9	2
90–99	8	1
100–149	11	3
150–199	12	. . .
200 and over	10	. . .
Total	256	256

Sources: Derived from official U.S. census data for 1950, 1960, and 1970.

table 2-10. The period used in the analysis of each technology is whichever proved most useful in explaining its adoption.

Another potential competitive influence on the decision to adopt a technology is the number or percentage of a hospital's competitors that already have it, a statistic that may represent local knowledge about the technology as well as the force of example. These percentages were used in the analysis of diffusion over time (chapters 3 and 4). In the analyses based on the 1975 survey, it was only possible to define a reasonable counterpart to this characteristic for intensive care beds (chapter 3). The discussion of these measures is left to chapters 3 and 4.

Financing

The ways in which hospitals raise money for investment projects have changed a great deal in the last ten to fifteen years. Philanthropy and government grants—or, for government-owned hospitals, appropriations —used to be the major sources of funds, with internal funds another important source. But partly because of the growth in third party payments, which count depreciation and interest as reimbursable expenses, the situation has changed and debt financing has emerged as the primary, and still growing, method for raising investment capital. In 1969 it already accounted for more than one-third of the capital raised by hospitals. By 1975 it had reached almost two-thirds, and Kelling and Williams predict that it will provide over 80 percent of investment financing by 1981.[21]

At the beginning of the study, an attempt was made to define separate measures for all the major sources of capital funds, in spite of the fact that the data in this area are few and far between and much of what is available is not very good. As the work progressed a few more deficiencies in the statistics came to light, and the cumulative effect of the deficiencies—in terms of erratic and meaningless results for these data in the statistical analysis—became clearer. The measures finally used represent a compromise between the ambitious plan laid down at the beginning and the skepticism that developed after longer acquaintance with the data. The discussion will outline briefly what was discarded and why and what was kept and why.

Three things were discarded: an attempt to use data from the Federal Reserve Board's survey of business loans as a proxy for the interest rate available on loans to hospitals; an attempt to represent the advantages offered by state legislation that makes it easier for private hospitals to issue tax-exempt bonds; and information about the federal Hill-Burton program of construction grants.

The first two were intended to represent debt financing directly. The Federal Reserve's survey of interest rates covers thirty-five financial centers. Although these data refer to all business loans made by banks, they were tried in the hope that they might represent the credit conditions available to hospitals; each SMSA was assigned the short-term interest rate, averaged over the years 1971–74, of the nearest financial center. The results were never sensible, and stratifying hospitals by the level of third party payment—on the hypothesis that their sensitivity to the interest rate

21. Lyman G. Van Nostrand, "Capital Financing for Health Facilities," *Public Health Reports*, vol. 92 (November–December 1977), pp. 499–507; Robert S. Kelling, Jr., and Paul C. Williams, "The Projected Response of the Capital Markets to Health Facilities Expenditures," in Gordon K. MacLeod and Mark Perlman, eds., *Health Care Capital: Competition and Control* (Ballinger, 1978), pp. 319–47. The percentages in the text refer to all hospital construction, not specifically to the construction or equipment associated with new technologies. New equipment can sometimes be acquired through leasing arrangements, but there is no information about how often this method is used or under what circumstances.

might differ with the extent to which the cost could be passed through to insurers—did not help. As will be discussed later, the insurance data have their own defects, and were a less-than-perfect instrument for the stratification.

The most reasonable conclusion was that the survey data were not, in fact, a good approximation of conditions in the market for hospital loans. As noted, the rates were those for all business loans, not hospital loans. The assignment to financial centers was necessarily arbitrary since it was based on geographical proximity rather than financial networks. But more important in this respect, the debt financing market is not as local as the Federal Reserve's use of thirty-five financial centers suggests it is. Large hospital bond issues are sold in what is effectively a national market, while even many smaller issues operate in regional markets that extend beyond the neighborhood of a single financial center. Thus the interest rate experiment was dropped from the analysis.

An American Hospital Association survey provided information about the existence and type of state legislation permitting hospitals to issue tax-exempt bonds.[22] Tax-exempt bonds carry a lower interest rate than other forms of debt, and thus hospitals in states with such legislation, especially states where the law has been in effect for quite a while, may find it easier to invest in new technologies. The year in which the legislation was passed was used to try to represent this influence.

But two problems gradually became apparent. Investigation of the tax-exempt bond market made it clear that there are many ways to confer tax-exempt status on a bond, and these differ enough in their ease and availability to create important distinctions among states. The survey did not give enough information about the legislation to permit these distinctions to be made. Even more disturbing, the years given for the legislation in the AHA survey are not consistent with information from other sources. Van Nostrand refers to Connecticut as the first state to pass a law making tax-exempt bonds easily available to private hospitals—in 1966—while the AHA survey lists a number of states, especially several southern ones, as having had legislation long before 1966.[23] Both statements may be true if the earlier legislation was of a much different and more limited kind than the later, but again this suggests that, at a minimum, a proper

22. American Hospital Association, Bureau of Fiscal Services, "Report on State Legislative Programs for the Capital Financing of Health Care Facilities" (AHA, April 1973); and updated tabulation, April 1977.

23. Van Nostrand, "Capital Financing for Health Facilities," pp. 502–03.

characterization of the effect of tax-exemption requires more information than was available from the survey.

Finally, data on Hill-Burton construction grants awarded to the states (the states distributed the money to individual applicants) were experimented with. The results were seldom statistically significant and seldom reasonable when they were significant. In this case, there was reason to question the relevance of the data rather than their accuracy. For most of the program's life, grants were awarded for the construction and renovation of hospitals, but the emphasis was on those in rural areas. After 1970 the emphasis shifted sharply away from hospitals altogether, toward clinics, laboratories, long-term care institutions, and the like. Thus, although measured by a single number, the grant money does not represent a single influence and may never have been particularly relevant to the adoption of technologies by metropolitan hospitals. In addition, it was particularly important to limit state data to those items for which there was a strong justification in order to minimize the problem of collinearity. The Hill-Burton data were omitted from the analysis.[24]

Data representing third party payment were retained from the early experiments. Although some of these data also suffer from serious defects, the decision to use them was based on the belief that the influence of third party payment is so important that it must have some empirical counterpart, however poor, in the analysis.[25] The analysis thus leaves out some factors that ideally should be included, because they are so poorly measured by the available data that including them introduces serious errors, and leaves in others, in spite of serious shortcomings in the data, because they are conceptually so important.

Third party payment is important because, as the major source of hospital revenues (about 90 percent of the total in the mid-1970s), it underlies the ability to generate internal funds for investment and to pay the interest costs on debt. Van Nostrand argues, in fact, that the choice between using debt and using internal revenues for investment is primarily one of timing—whether the hospital prefers to spend its money first and be reimbursed or get the money first before spending it.

24. The state data can take on only forty-seven separate values and thus do not have the scope for independent variation that the SMSA or hospital data have. The forty-seven include the District of Columbia and all of the states except Alaska, Hawaii, Vermont, and Wyoming. There are no SMSAs in the last two.
25. The results for each technology are, however, presented both with and without the data for third party payment.

But more important, of course, very high levels of third party payment remove the financial constraints from hospitals altogether. As third party payment rises toward these levels, hospitals are increasingly able to pursue investment projects—including investment in new technologies—without concern for costs. Nominal financial restraints such as the interest rate on debt lose their meaning and fade into insignificance because they can simply be passed on to third party payers. Thus as third party payment increases, the adoption of technologies will proceed more rapidly and be more extensive. With such important effects to be measured, it is especially unfortunate that the available data—especially the historical data—are so inadequate.

The first two items of data used to represent third party payment are the percentage of the population covered by hospital insurance in 1963, and the growth in that percentage between 1961 and 1971.[26] The primary defect of both items is that the data are available only at the level of the state, not the SMSA. This means that sizable differences between hospital markets are hidden under a single state average that may not represent the situation in most SMSAs. Actually, the growth in insurance does incorporate a little information about each SMSA. It was calculated by first adding the percentage of the state population that was both under sixty-five years of age and covered by hospital insurance in 1971, and the percentage of the SMSA's population that was sixty-five years or older in 1970 (Medicare covers virtually all of this group). The percentage of the state population with hospital insurance in 1961 was then subtracted from this sum and the difference was expressed as a percentage of the 1961 level. Thus the growth rate over the decade is a hybrid, unique to the SMSA but based primarily on state data.

The insurance data are reported by the insured person's state of employment rather than state of residence. It is not clear which state better matches patterns of hospital use, but the population data used to calculate the percentages are based on state of residence, and the disagreement in this respect between the two sets of data makes the percentages still

26. The use of a 1963 base and a 1961–71 growth rate is an accident. The 1963 data were the earliest kept on the condensed data file, but the growth between 1963 and 1973 could not be computed because the 1973 data were reported by state of residence, rather than state of employment, making them incompatible with the earlier years. The growth between 1961 and 1971 was calculated instead and added to the file, but the 1961 data were not. It did not seem worthwhile to correct this oversight since the 1961 and 1963 data are virtually identical for statistical purposes; the correlation between them is 0.982.

Table 2-11. Distributions of States and Standard Metropolitan Statistical Areas by Percent of Population with Hospital Insurance, 1963

Percent of population with hospital insurance	Number of states[a]	Number of SMSAs[b]
45–49	2	3
50–54	1	2
55–59	4	13
60–64	5	29
65–69	6	53
70–74	9	42
75–79	6	25
80–84	7	39
85–89	4	39
90 and over	3	11
Total	47	256

Sources: State data on number of people with hospital insurance from Health Insurance Institute, *Source Book of Health Insurance Data, 1964–65* (HII, n.d.); state populations from U.S. Bureau of the Census, *Statistical Abstract of the United States, 1970* (GPO, 1970).

a. Includes the District of Columbia and excludes Wyoming and Vermont, which have no SMSAs, and Alaska and Hawaii.

b. SMSAs are classified on the basis of the percent for the state in which the largest portion of the SMSA population lives.

more imperfect. It would also have been better to have the percentage of hospital costs covered rather than the percentage of people with insurance, but these data were available only for later years (still at the state level). The period from the early 1960s to the early 1970s was preferable on conceptual grounds both for the analysis of the years 1961–75 and for the analysis of the 1975 hospital data, since most of the technologies examined in the latter case also spread during the 1960s.[27] Finally, the data ignore the introduction of Medicaid and there was no way to correct for this.

Both measures show considerable variation, although one can only speculate about the accuracy of this variation or how much more may exist within states (tables 2-11 and 2-12). Since the data are primarily state data, both tables show the distributions for states as well as SMSAs. The state distribution gives the most accurate picture of the extent of variation in the data, and the SMSA distribution translates this into numbers of SMSAs.

These two items were supplemented by a third—the percentage of hospital costs in each SMSA paid by Medicare in 1971. Logically, this

27. Experiments with data for later years, which frequently produced erratic and unreasonable results, support this preference.

Table 2-12. Distributions of States and Standard Metropolitan Statistical Areas by Growth in Proportion of Population with Hospital Insurance, 1961-71

Percent growth in population with hospital insurance[a]	Number of states[b]	Number of SMSAs
Negative	1	2
0–9	5	19
10–19	13	85
20–29	11	60
30–39	5	41
40–49	6	26
50–59	4	13
60–69	2	9
70–79	0	1
Total	47	256

Sources: State data on number of people with hospital insurance in 1961 from Health Insurance Institute, *Source Book of Health Insurance Data, 1962–63* (HII, n.d.); number of people under sixty-five years with hospital insurance in 1971, ibid., *1972–73;* number of people in each SMSA sixty-five years or older from official 1970 census data; population data are from various issues of Bureau of the Census, *Statistical Abstract,* and the 1970 census.

a. This growth is calculated as (1) the proportion of the population with hospital insurance in 1971 (calculated for each SMSA as the proportion of the state population that was both under sixty-five years and covered by hospital insurance, plus the proportion of the SMSA's population that was sixty-five or older in 1970 and thus covered by Medicare) minus (2) the proportion with insurance in 1961 (state data), (3) the difference between 1 and 2 taken as a percent of the 1961 level.

b. Classified by the average for all the SMSAs in the state.

does not belong in the analysis, because Medicare is already accounted for in the 1961–71 growth rate. But empirically the data available are so much better than any other data on financing, particularly in being available at the level of the SMSA, that they were included in the hope of capturing some of the differences between SMSAs that the state data fail to capture.

The Medicare data are not, however, without a few difficulties of their own. Both the numerator and the denominator are subject to problems that cause them to be underestimated. The numerator, Medicare reimbursements, is based on interim payments made during the calendar year; when all the necessary adjustments are made at the end of the year, the final payments always turn out to be higher.[28] The denominator, short-term hospital costs in the SMSA, refers to a fiscal year that ends in September for most hospitals and even earlier for some;[29] the steady growth of hospital costs guarantees that this number is somewhat less than costs

28. Information provided by the Social Security Administration.

29. *Hospitals, Journal of the American Hospital Association,* vol. 45 (August 1, 1971), Guide Issue, pt. 2, and preceding annual guide issues; *American Hospital Association, Hospital Statistics,* annual.

for the year ending in December. But it seems reasonable to expect that these understatements approximately cancel.

There is an additional problem with the numerator, however, that results in its being overstated relative to the denominator. Reimbursements under the hospital insurance part (part A) of the Medicare program include payments to long-term hospitals and extended-care facilities as well as payments to short-term hospitals. By 1971, due to a deliberate policy of cutting back on the approval of claims of extended-care facilities, these payments had been reduced to 5 percent of the total paid nationally under part A.[30] Nonetheless, they were undoubtedly much more important than this in some SMSAs, and the percentage of hospital costs paid by Medicare may be significantly overstated as a result. This is particularly likely to be a problem for the SMSAs with the highest calculated percentages.

In 1971 Medicare paid, on average, about 20 percent of all short-term hospital costs.[31] Table 2-13 shows that the percentages paid in the 256 SMSAs vary considerably around the average. Most SMSAs fall between 10 and 30 percent, a wide range to start with, but seven fall below 10 percent and twenty-seven fall above 30 percent. In large part, of course, this reflects the variability across SMSAs in the percentage of elderly people in the population. Nationally, people sixty-five years or older account for 10 percent of the population and more than 25 percent of all hospital costs.[32] As a first approximation then, an SMSA with, say, 20 percent of its population sixty-five years or older could expect to have Medicare pay as much as 50 percent of its hospital costs. Consistent with this reasoning, the four SMSAs with Medicare shares of more than 45 percent are all in Florida.

Two final and very important points must be made about these data. First, even at the beginning of the period the level of third party payment was high. Table 2-11 shows that in only three states was less than 55 percent of the population covered in 1963, and these states had fewer than

30. *Social Security Bulletin,* vol. 36 (September 1973), tables M-19 and M-20.
31. Estimate based on data reported in Barbara S. Cooper, Nancy L. Worthington, and Mary F. McGee, *Compendium of National Health Expenditures Data,* Social Security Administration, DHEW pub. (SSA) 76-11927 (GPO, 1976).
32. Marjorie Smith Mueller and Robert M. Gibson, "Age Differences in Health Care Spending, Fiscal Year 1975," *Social Security Bulletin,* vol. 39 (June 1976), pp. 18–19.

Table 2-13. Distribution of Standard Metropolitan Statistical Areas by Percent of Hospital Costs Paid by Medicare, 1971

Percent of hospital costs paid by Medicare	Number of SMSAs
0–4	2
5–9	5
10–14	20
15–19	72
20–24	83
25–29	47
30–34	14
35–39	6
40–44	3
45–49	2
50 and over	2
Total	256

Sources: Medicare data from Social Security Administration, *Medicare: Health Insurance for the Aged: Amounts Reimbursed, by State and County, 1971* (SSA, Office of Research and Statistics, 1973); total expenses for nonfederal short-term hospitals from AHA's 1971 survey of hospitals. Hospital expenses, which were adjusted to take account of hospitals that did not fill in this part of the survey questionnaire, are for the fiscal year that ended in the year of the survey. Most hospitals end their fiscal year on September 30.

50 metropolitan hospitals among them in 1975. Thus, even if the data were perfect, the statistical analysis could only show the effects of additions to an already high level of third party payment. It could not show the important changes already brought about by the initial level or, as a consequence, what the situation would be with little or no third party payment.

Second, it cannot be emphasized too strongly that these data are included in the analysis, not because they represent third party payment well, but because they are all there is and third party payment is too important to omit entirely. Given their deficiencies, it is not reasonable to expect them to produce much evidence about the effect of third party payment—in fact, they do not—and what they do produce cannot be considered authoritative. The main weight of the evidence concerning third party payment in this study thus comes from the case studies, not the statistical analysis. As discussed in chapter 1, the case studies demonstrate the consequences that follow when hospitals are freed from economic restraints: large investments have been and are being made, even though the benefits of the technologies—sometimes in total, sometimes in some of their major applications—are small, or even questionable.

Regulation

The federal government introduced two programs in the middle 1960s, the regional medical program and the comprehensive health planning program, with the intention of influencing the use of resources in medical care and, to a greater or lesser extent, their use in the form of new technologies. One by one, through the latter half of the 1960s, and then in groups in the early 1970s, the states added another program—certificate-of-need reviews of investment projects proposed by hospitals. Fortunately, reasonably good data exist for all three programs.[33]

The purpose of the regional medical program (RMP) was to promote the faster and more extensive diffusion of new technologies. Passed in 1965 and entirely federally funded, the legislation initially directed that funds be concentrated on technologies for the treatment of heart disease, cancer, and stroke. With coronary care units just getting started (see chapter 3), many regional programs enthusiastically committed funds to train nurses and physicians in coronary care and other even newer uses for intensive care, such as for stroke. Technologies for the treatment of cancer were not in a state that made it so easy to settle on an approach and these projects developed more slowly. Kidney disease was added to the program's charge by the amendments of 1970 and a technology—renal dialysis—was ready and waiting for support; but after only a year or two to plan projects, the RMP became embroiled in a battle for survival it finally lost in 1975. Judging from the published accounts of what the regional programs did during their lifetimes, if RMPs had an important effect on any technology, it was on intensive care. Renal dialysis is a less likely but still obvious possibility.[34]

The effect of the RMP can be tested by distinguishing among the RMP regions according to the amount of money at their disposal. Fifty-one program regions both received money during the years 1967–74 and contained one or more SMSAs (table 2-14). To represent the influence the programs might have had on individual hospitals, the funds are divided by the number of nonfederal short-term hospitals in an RMP area and the

33. These programs are discussed again, in another context and at greater length, in chapter 6.

34. Nancy Kay, "The Regional Medical Programs: Contributions to Technological Diffusion" (unpublished paper available from author).

Table 2-14. Distributions of Regional Medical Program Areas and Standard Metropolitan Statistical Areas by Program Dollars per Hospital, 1967–74

RMP dollars	Number of SMSAs	Number of RMP areas
25,000–49,999	35	4
50,000–99,999	95	18
100,000–149,999	92	16
150,000–199,999	13	4
200,000–299,999	12	5
300,000–399,999	9	4
Total	256	51

Sources: Data on total funds awarded 1967–74 provided by the Department of Health, Education, and Welfare. The number of nonfederal short-term hospitals in RMP areas in 1969 based on AHA's 1969 survey of hospitals and on county definitions of RMP areas provided by HEW.

resulting average is assigned to each SMSA in that area. The range of funds per hospital is fairly wide—twenty-two RMP areas, containing 130 SMSAs, received less than $100,000 per hospital over the eight years, while twenty-nine RMP areas, with 126 SMSAs among them, received $100,000 or more.

The comprehensive health planning (CHP) program was passed a year later, in 1966. Aimed at encouraging the regional planning of medical resources, it financed planning agencies at two levels—states and smaller areas within states. These agencies were given so little guidance by the legislation that their influence could have been exerted either toward promoting the diffusion of technologies or toward restraining it, or even both, depending on the technology and the preferences of the particular agency. They were given no powers, other than those inherent in their limited funds, to pursue their objectives.

The area agencies got only part of their funds from the federal government. By law it could provide no more than 75 percent of the total, and it usually provided less—in 1972, for example, the federal share averaged 54 percent and ranged from 25 to 75 percent.[35] Thus the distribution of federal funds per hospital across SMSAs (table 2-15) may not accurately reflect the distribution of total funds. Even so, it is clear that the area CHP agencies had much less money than the regional medical programs, and their influence could reasonably be expected to be commensurately less.

35. *Comprehensive Health Planning as Carried out by State and Areawide Agencies in Three States,* Report to the Congress by the Comptroller General of the United States (U.S. General Accounting Office, 1974), p. 8.

Table 2-15. Distributions of Standard Metropolitan Statistical Areas by Area Comprehensive Health Planning Dollars per Hospital, 1968–72

Area CHP dollars	Number of SMSAs	Number of unduplicated SMSAs[a]
0	81	...
1–499	0	...
500–999	4	3
1,000–4,999	37	28
5,000–9,999	40	34
10,000–14,999	40	31
15,000–24,999	31	27
25,000 and over	23	20
Total	256	143

Sources: Data on funds awarded 1968–72 provided by the Department of Health, Education, and Welfare. Number of nonfederal short-term hospitals in CHP areas in 1969 based on American Hospital Association's 1969 survey of hospitals. The county definitions of CHP areas were taken from Jeannette Fitzwilliams, *A Profile of U.S. Comprehensive Health Planning Areas*, Agricultural Economic Report 339 (Economic Research Service, 1976); ibid., *Supplemental Data: Characteristics and County Composition of CHP Areas, Regions II, III, and V* (ERS, n.d.); ibid, *Region IV;* ibid., *Regions VI, IX, and X;* and ibid., *Regions VII and VIII.*

a. Some area CHP agencies included two or three SMSAs in their jurisdictions. This column excludes the second, or second and third, SMSAs from the count and thus gives the number of distinct values for funds per hospital. This is not the same as the number of CHP areas, because some SMSAs encompass more than one such area.

The CHP agencies at both the area and state levels became involved in promoting the passage, during the late 1960s and early 1970s, of certificate-of-need laws in the states (table 2-16). These laws—which require a state agency to approve investment projects proposed by hospitals (see chapter 6)—gave many of the CHPs in the affected states their first taste of power, because they were consulted in the review process. Certificate-of-need reviews were intended to prevent "unnecessary duplication" of facilities and the construction of "too many" hospital beds. As with the regional medical and comprehensive health planning programs, there is no reason to believe that, if certificate-of-need has had an effect, that effect has been uniform; which technologies were affected, and how, would depend on which were considered by the reviewers to be worthy of further expansion and which were considered to be overexpanded already. But in contrast to the RMP literature, the published literature about the CHP program and certificate-of-need reviews does not suggest anything about these perceptions of different technologies.

The statistical analysis distinguishes between states with the earliest laws (1965–69) and states with laws that became effective during the years 1970 to 1973, and it groups states with laws passed later together with those still without laws at the end of 1975, on the supposition that a

Table 2-16. Distributions of States and Standard Metropolitan Statistical Areas by Year Certificate-of-Need Legislation Became Effective

Year	Number of states	Number of SMSAs[a]
1965	1	10
1966	0	0
1967	0	0
1968	1	1
1969	1	4
1970	2	19
1971	8	36
1972	6	24
1973	4	27
1974[b]	2	15
1975[b]	3	31
After 1975 or no legislation	19[c]	89
Total	47[d]	256

Sources: Data for 1973 and earlier provided by David S. Salkever, School of Hygiene and Public Health, Johns Hopkins University; data for 1974 and 1975 provided by Department of Health, Education, and Welfare, Office of Health Maintenance Organizations.

a. For the purposes of this tabulation, SMSAs that cross state boundaries are counted only once and are assigned the year of the state that accounts for the largest portion of their population.

b. Year legislation was enacted rather than year it went into effect.

c. Oklahoma is counted as not having a certificate-of-need law because its law, passed in 1971, covers only nursing homes.

d. Excludes Vermont and Wyoming, which have no SMSAs.

law passed after 1973 could not have had time to influence whether a hospital had a particular technology in 1975. Only three states had laws in effect between 1965 and 1969—New York, Connecticut, and Rhode Island. Since New York has more SMSAs than the others, and many more hospitals, the results for this group are dominated by New York's policies and experience.

Data on the federal funds paid to state CHP agencies were also available. But the history of the program gives no reason to believe that these agencies had any important way of influencing technological diffusion other than through certificate-of-need reviews. Thus to keep the number of state variables to a minimum, these data were left out of the analysis.[36]

Summary

This chapter outlines a number of factors that may influence a hospital in its decision to adopt a new technology and discusses the data used to

36. In most states, the funds averaged less than $10,000 per hospital over fiscal years 1967–72.

represent these factors in the statistical analysis. The analysis of these data can help to answer some interesting questions about why certain hospitals adopt particular technologies and why others do not. Are the characteristics of patients or of their doctors given greater weight in hospitals' decisions? How important is the influence of medical schools? What part does the competitive structure of the market play? What have been the effects of government intervention through the regional medical program, the comprehensive health planning program, and state certificate-of-need laws? The analyses presented in chapters 3, 4, and 5 examine these factors.

chapter three Intensive Care

If one technology could be said to be the hallmark of the modern hospital, it is the intensive care unit. Intensive care was and is in large part an organizational innovation, built on the simple idea that critically ill patients need close observation, constant nursing, and quick action in a crisis, and that the most efficient way to provide this kind of care is not to disperse these patients throughout the wards, but to bring them together in one place with the most sophisticated equipment and highly trained people in the hospital. Historically, intensive care has been both the natural consequence of new methods of patient monitoring and life support and the stimulus for their invention.

It first appeared about the time of the Second World War in the form of the postoperative recovery room. Located near the operating rooms, the recovery room is a place where patients who have just undergone surgery are cared for until they have come safely through the anesthesia and the immediate aftereffects of the surgery itself.[1] In 1951, only about 20 percent of all community hospitals with 100 beds or more had recovery rooms. In the manner typical of hospital technologies, recovery rooms spread first and fastest through the largest hospitals and more slowly through successively smaller ones (figure 3-1).[2] By the early 1960s virtually all hospitals of more than 100 beds reported recovery rooms. Their adoption is not yet complete among hospitals with fewer than 100 beds, but even so, 70 percent of these hospitals had recovery rooms in 1976, up from only about 5 percent in 1951.

1. Carl G. Schowengerdt, "The Recovery Room," in William H. L. Dornette, ed., *Clinical Anesthesia,* vol. 9/2, 3: *Monitoring in Anesthesia* (Philadelphia: F. A. Davis, 1973), pp. 363–70; Carl E. Wasmuth, "The Anesthesiologist and the Intensive Care Unit," *International Anesthesiology Clinics,* vol. 11 (Winter 1973), pp. 117–40.

2. Since the pattern of adoption sometimes varies with the control of the hospital as well as with its size, figure 3-1 charts private nonprofit hospitals rather than all community hospitals.

41

Figure 3-1. Percent of Private Nonprofit Hospitals with Postoperative Recovery Rooms, 1953–76, and Intensive Care Units, 1958–76[a], by Size of Hospital

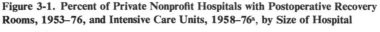
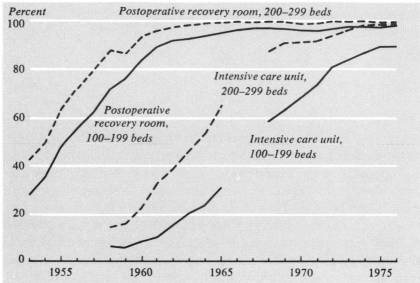

Sources: *Hospitals, Journal of the American Hospital Association*, vol. 45 (August 1, 1971), Guide Issue, pt. 2 and selected preceding annual guide issues; *Hospital Statistics*, selected annual issues.

a. Gaps in the lines reflect years in which the facility was omitted from the survey.

With its strong appeal to common sense, the philosophy of intensive care was bound to find wider application. The average hospital sees many patients during the course of a year who are in critical condition. Many of them are suffering from heart attacks or other coronary conditions. Suicide attempts, severe asthma, gastrointestinal bleeding, acute kidney or liver failure, and other such conditions appear frequently. The development of new and more extensive types of surgery, particularly open-heart surgery, created a need for care of a much higher order and over a much longer period than required by the usual surgical patient. The mixed intensive care unit (ICU), designed to accommodate all these patients, followed the recovery room by about a decade.[3]

3. Douglas G. Carroll, "Patterns of Medical Care in a Municipal Hospital Intensive Care Unit: Convenience or Necessity?" *Maryland State Medical Journal*, vol. 20 (January 1971), pp. 89–94; J. V. Collins, T. R. Evans, and T. J. H. Clark, "Basic Equipment for Medical Intensive-Care Units," *Lancet*, vol. 1, no. 7693 (February 6, 1971), pp. 285–87; Paul F. Griner, "Treatment of Acute Pulmonary Edema: Conventional or Intensive Care?" *Annals of Internal Medicine*, vol. 77 (October 1972), pp. 501–06; and Paul F. Griner, "Medical Intensive Care in the Teaching Hospital: Costs Versus Benefits: The Need for an Assessment," *Annals of Internal Medicine*, vol. 78 (April 1973), pp. 581–85.

In 1958, the first year the American Hospital Association included the mixed ICU in its survey, its diffusion was still rather limited. Only about 25 percent of the largest community hospitals (300 or more beds) reported one. The mixed ICU proved just as popular as the recovery room, and by 1976 nearly all community hospitals with 200 beds or more reported one, not quite 90 percent of hospitals with 100 through 199 beds, and almost 50 percent of those with still fewer beds. The trends show that the ICU is still spreading among hospitals in the two smallest size groups.

As new equipment and techniques for treating patients with heart conditions appeared—the defibrillator, the pacemaker, anticoagulant therapy, and others—it became inevitable that a new unit would be created specifically for these patients.[4] In 1962, the first coronary care units (CCUs) were established independently, and almost simultaneously, in at least three urban medical centers in North America. Evidence was accumulating to show that irregularities in heart rhythm often preceded more serious crises in the coronary patient, and the hope was that by watching closely for these irregularities and trying to correct them at once, the staff of the unit could reduce the death rate from heart attacks. By 1976 the vast majority of hospitals with 300 or more beds had separate CCUs for heart patients. So did 57 percent of community hospitals with 200 through 299 beds, 29 percent of those with 100 through 199 beds, and even 18 percent of those with fewer than 100 beds. Some hospitals had gone a step further and spun off intermediate coronary care units (ICCUs) for patients believed to need the attention of people trained in the treatment of heart conditions, but not as much attention as provided in the CCU.[5]

The refinement and extension of the intensive care philosophy has not stopped with coronary units. The larger the hospital, the more likely it is to have additional units and subunits: separate units for medical and surgical patients, stroke units, respiratory units, renal units, burn units, neonatal units for the intensive care of newborns, pediatric units. The future no doubt holds still others. But for the present the recovery room,

4. T. D. V. Lawrie, "Advances in the Treatment of Cardiovascular Disease," *Practitioner,* vol. 203 (October 1969), pp. 460–67; Thomas Killip and John T. Kimball, "A Survey of the Coronary Care Unit: Concept and Results," *Progress in Cardiovascular Diseases,* vol. 11 (July 1968), pp. 45–52.

5. Julian Friedan and Jerome A. Cooper, "The Role of the Intermediate Cardiac Care Unit," *Journal of the American Medical Association,* vol. 235 (February 23, 1976), pp. 816–18.

the mixed intensive care unit, and perhaps a separate coronary unit (or subunit within the mixed ICU) represent the bulk of intensive care.

Table 3-1 shows the distributions of ICU and CCU beds by region. The table includes the beds in federal as well as nonfederal hospitals and relates them to the population and to total hospital beds. (This study concerns itself almost exclusively with nonfederal hospitals, but it would be misleading to compare only the facilities in these hospitals with the total population of a region, some of whom do have access to federal facilities.) The distribution is surprisingly uniform. The number of beds per 10,000 population in the best endowed regions, the Pacific and West North Central states, is only about 25 percent greater than the number in the two least endowed, the Middle Atlantic and East North Central states (two regions that one is not used to finding at the low end of any scale). The somewhat greater disparity in the proportion of all hospital beds committed to intensive care is due to the fact that all beds are less uniformly distributed than are intensive care beds.

At the less aggregated level of the SMSA, there is, of course, considerably more variation, but each of the 255 metropolitan areas in the 1975 AHA survey has at least one hospital with an ICU or CCU (table 3-2). The areas at either extreme of the distribution are largely those one would

Table 3-1. Distributions of Intensive Care and Coronary Care Beds, by Region, 1976

| | Number of intensive care and coronary care beds | | |
| | | Per 10,000 | Per 100 |
Region	Total	population	hospital beds
New England	2,928	2.4	5.3
Middle Atlantic	8,213	2.2	4.5
South Atlantic	7,894	2.3	4.8
East North Central	8,805	2.2	4.3
East South Central	3,180	2.3	4.4
West North Central	4,731	2.8	4.5
West South Central	5,063	2.4	4.6
Mountain	2,253	2.3	5.2
Pacific	8,003	2.8	6.6
United States	51,070	2.4	4.8

Sources: Intensive care and coronary care beds (all hospitals) and hospital beds in federal general and nonfederal short-term hospitals, American Hospital Association, *Hospital Statistics, 1977 Edition* (AHA, 1977); population data, provisional estimates for July 1976, Bureau of the Census, *Current Population Reports*, series P-25, no. 642, "Revised 1975 and Provisional 1976 Estimates of the Population of States, and Components of Change, 1970 to 1976" (Government Printing Office, 1976).

Table 3-2. Distributions of Standard Metropolitan Statistical Areas by Percent of Beds in Intensive Care and Coronary Care Units in Short-Term Hospitals, 1975

Percent of beds in intensive care and coronary care units	Number of SMSAs by type of hospital	
	Federal and nonfederal hospitals	Nonfederal hospitals
1.0–1.9	3	3
2.0–2.9	11	10
3.0–3.9	41	36
4.0–4.9	82	79
5.0–5.9	71	67
6.0–6.9	33	37
7.0–7.9	8	16
8.0–8.9	6	6
9.0–9.9	0	1
All	255	255

Source: Derived from the American Hospital Association's 1975 survey of hospitals.

expect to find. At the low end, most of the SMSAs are small and located in the South or the Middle West. At the high end, there are quite a few cities in California (as table 3-1 shows, a high percentage of the Pacific region's hospital beds are in intensive care), a sprinkling of major medical centers (New Haven, Connecticut, and Rochester, Minnesota), several cities in Florida, and a few cities for which the explanation is not so immediately obvious (Great Falls, Montana, for example, or Waco, Texas).

Intensive care has changed the character of hospitals and hospital care in the last twenty-five years. Virtually by definition, it involves using more of everything: more space; more equipment (and more sophisticated equipment); more laboratory tests; and more labor, especially nursing time. Its use of resources has been a major element in the growth of hospital costs.[6]

The ratio of nurses to patients depends on how seriously ill the patients in the unit tend to be. The Society for Critical Care Medicine recommends one specially trained nurse per patient per eight-hour shift,[7] but

6. For a detailed account of the resources used to provide intensive care, see Louise B. Russell and Carol S. Burke, *Technological Diffusion in the Hospital Sector,* prepared for the National Science Foundation (National Planning Association, October 1975; available from the National Technical Information Service, report no. PB 245 642/AS), chap. 3.

7. "Guidelines for Organization of Critical Care Units," *Journal of the American Medical Association,* vol. 222 (December 18, 1972), pp. 1532–35.

others have found that this ratio is only necessary for very seriously ill patients, a minority in any ICU. On average, intensive care units use almost three times as many nursing hours per patient day as general medical and surgical wards do.[8] In addition to nurses, who make up the bulk of an ICU's staff, units employ medical residents, equipment technicians, respiratory therapists, lab technicians, computer programmers, clerical help, and other supporting staff in greater numbers than do general wards.[9]

The list of equipment in an intensive care unit is equally long. In most units an electrocardiograph for each patient is standard. X-rays and lab tests—blood-gas analyses to check on respiration, for example—are done much more frequently in the ICU than in the wards, and many units have their own labs and X-ray equipment for these procedures. In especially sophisticated units, closed-circuit television and computers help with the monitoring. Pacemakers, defibrillators (machines that deliver electrical impulses to the heart), ventilators (machines that maintain the patient's breathing), kidney dialysis machines, and other therapeutic and life-support equipment are ready to be brought into use.[10]

Four beds is the smallest size considered economic for a unit, and if more than twelve or fifteen beds are needed, a second unit is usually established. Because of the sicker patients, the larger staff, and the larger amount of equipment, intensive care uses more space per bed than does ward care. All but the smallest units are largely self-contained, with their own nursing stations, offices, conference rooms, waiting rooms, laboratories, storage areas, and other "overhead" facilities.[11]

---

8. A recent survey reports that, in hospitals with fifty or more beds, nursing time averaged sixteen to seventeen hours per patient day in the ICU, against less than six hours in the wards. William A. Michela, "Administrative Profiles: Employee Fringe Benefits," *Hospitals, Journal of the American Hospital Association,* vol. 50 (November 1, 1976), p. 68.

9. "Guidelines for Organization of Critical Care Units"; "Standards for Special Care Units: Guidelines for Organization, Staffing, and Costs," *Modern Hospital,* vol. 118 (January 1972), pp. 83–87.

10. Paul F. Griner and Benjamin Liptzin, "Use of the Laboratory in a Teaching Hospital: Implications for Patient Care, Education, and Hospital Costs," *Annals of Internal Medicine,* vol. 75 (August 1971), pp. 157–63; "Guidelines for Organization of Critical Care Units"; G. Vourc'h and others, "Surgical Intensive Care," *British Journal of Surgery,* vol. 54 (1967), Supplement, pp. 459–62; Per Erik Wiklund, "Intensive Care Units: Design, Location, Staffing Ancillary Areas, Equipment," *Anesthesiology,* vol. 31 (August 1969), pp. 122–36.

11. "Guidelines for Organization of Critical Care Units"; Wiklund, "Intensive Care Units"; Dorothy M. Wylie, "Designing an Intensive Care Unit," *Hospital Administration in Canada,* vol. 14 (May 1972), pp. 68–71.

Intensive care calls on so many other facilities in the hospital and is involved with so many kinds of treatment, some of which might be impossible without it, that it is difficult to estimate all the costs associated with it. But even a partial accounting makes it clear that they are very high.

Data for the University of Rochester's Medical Center show that, in one recent year, the operating costs of intensive care—including salaries, equipment costs, indirect costs, and X-ray and laboratory procedures— were $400 per day, more than 3.6 times the ward cost of $110.[12] At the Massachusetts General Hospital, the average charge per day in the surgical ICU was estimated at $761 for 1970, about 4.1 times the $187 average for ward care.[13] A Pittsburgh hospital contrasts fiscal 1970 costs of $111 and $114 per day in the mixed intensive and coronary care units, with $41 per day in conventional wards, for ratios of 2.7:1 and 2.8:1, respectively.[14] These figures probably understate the cost of intensive care relative to ward care, since they appear to exclude laboratory, X-ray, and other ancillary costs. A British study also reports that the cost of intensive care is about three times that of ward care.[15]

The evidence suggests, then, that the cost of a day in an ICU can be conservatively estimated at three times the cost of a day on the wards. Using this ratio, and the fact that, in 1976, 5.2 of every 100 beds in community hospitals were in intensive or coronary care units, it is possible to calculate the contribution of intensive care to hospital costs in more aggregate terms. If all hospital beds were in wards, the daily cost of care would be the cost of ward care. In reality, of course, the cost of a day in the hospital is an average of intensive care and ward costs. Assuming that days of care are proportional to numbers of beds, this average can be expressed as:

average cost per hospital day

$$= \frac{(3 \times \text{ward cost per day} \times \text{IC beds}) + (\text{ward cost per day} \times \text{ward beds})}{\text{total beds}}$$

12. Griner, "Medical Intensive Care in the Teaching Hospital." (The article does not give the exact year for the cost data.)

13. Joseph M. Civetta, "The Inverse Relationship Between Cost and Survival," *Journal of Surgical Research,* vol. 14 (March 1973), pp. 265–69.

14. "Standards for Special Care Units."

15. A. A. Sissouras and B. Moores, "Cost Analysis of a System of Intensive Coronary Care Services (Coronary and Mobile Units)," *Hospital and Health Services Review,* vol. 71 (January 1975), pp. 12–16.

The terms in this formula can be rearranged to express the ratio of average cost to ward cost per day as a function of the division of hospital beds between intensive care units and wards:

$$\frac{\text{average cost per hospital day}}{\text{ward cost per day}} = 3 \times \frac{\text{IC beds}}{\text{total beds}} + \frac{\text{ward beds}}{\text{total beds}}.$$

With intensive care beds accounting for 5.2 percent of total hospital beds and ward beds for the remaining 94.8 percent, the formula shows that the cost per hospital day was more than 10 percent higher in 1976 than it would have been had all hospital beds been in wards. In dollar terms, the cost per hospital day could have been $143 in 1976 instead of the $158 actually recorded. Since the three-to-one ratio is conservative, and since recovery room beds are not included in the count of intensive care beds, this estimate is more likely to underestimate than to overestimate intensive care's contribution to hospital costs.

The formula used to produce this estimate does not allow for the possibility that ward costs might be considerably higher if the critically ill patients admitted to intensive care were kept on the wards instead. It may be that the greater use of nursing time, lab tests, and so on, per patient in intensive care is offset by reductions in their use in the ward, because the patients left on the wards are not as sick. If this is true, intensive care represents a rearrangement of the resources used by hospitals, rather than an increase.

This hypothesis cannot be rejected, but the few fragments of evidence available do not support it. Paul F. Griner observes that the establishment of an ICU at the University of Rochester Medical Center was not followed by any reduction in the staff of the wards.[16] In another study, he reports that patients with acute pulmonary edema who were admitted to intensive care for some portion of their stay averaged 5.4 blood-gas analyses per stay, compared with 0.65 analysis for ward patients with the same diagnosis and 0.55 analysis for *all* patients with that diagnosis in the year prior to the opening of the ICU.[17] And an article about intensive care at Peter Bent Brigham Hospital notes that, although the hospital's total number of beds grew only slightly between 1960 and 1971, the total number of employees grew from 700 to 1,700, with the largest increases following the

16. Griner, "Medical Intensive Care in the Teaching Hospital."
17. Griner, "Treatment of Acute Pulmonary Edema."

establishment of mixed and coronary care units.[18] All three studies contradict the argument that intensive care is simply a rearrangement of patients and hospital resources.

Another challenge is, So what if it is expensive? If it does a lot of good, it is probably well worth the money. The subject of the benefits of intensive care deserves a section of its own, both for what it shows about intensive care and for what it shows about the difficulties of measuring the benefits of any kind of medical care. That discussion will be postponed to the end of the chapter. The next two sections take up the statistical analysis of the speed with which hospitals adopted intensive care units over the years 1961–75 and the number of intensive care beds they reported in 1975.

The Statistical Analysis:
The Diffusion of Intensive Care, 1961–75

As the preceding section describes, the diffusion of intensive care took place primarily during the 1960s and the first half of the 1970s. Of the 2,770 metropolitan hospitals that responded to the AHA survey in at least ten of the fifteen years between 1961 and 1975—the years for which the surveys are available on tape—1,705, distributed across 246 SMSAs, reported that they established either a mixed ICU or a CCU during the period. This section presents a statistical analysis of the differences in the lengths of time it took hospitals to adopt this technology.

The length of time is measured by the number of years from the first survey, 1961, until the hospital reported either an ICU or a CCU. As the earlier discussion brought out, the dividing line between the two can be unclear since hospitals that have a mixed ICU but not a separate CCU admit patients with heart conditions to the ICU. In fact, during the late 1960s, when the survey first started asking about separate CCUs, there was considerable confusion in the responses: some hospitals would report one year that they had a CCU but no ICU, the next year that they had an ICU but no CCU. For this analysis, the information about both units was

18. Alfred Morgan, Carolyn Daly, and Benjamin J. Murawski, "Dollar and Human Costs of Intensive Care," *Journal of Surgical Research,* vol. 14 (May 1973), pp. 441–48.

Table 3-3. Number and Percent of Study Hospitals Adopting Intensive Care Units, by Year of Adoption and Size of Hospital, 1962–75

	Hospitals	
Factor	Number	Percent
Year of adoption		
1962	93	5.5
1963	143	8.4
1964	132	7.7
1965	186	10.9
1966[a]	n.a.	n.a.
1967[a]	n.a.	n.a.
1968	534	31.3
1969	218	12.8
1970	106	6.2
1971	104	6.1
1972	67	3.9
1973	52	3.0
1974	34	2.0
1975	36	2.1
Total	1,705	100.0
Beds in hospital[b]		
Under 100	454	26.6
100–199	577	33.8
200–299	328	19.2
300 and over	346	20.3
Total	1,705	100.0

Sources: AHA's surveys of hospitals, 1961 through 1975 (1961 data not included in the table, because adoptions in 1961 could not be distinguished from those in earlier years); metropolitan hospitals that responded to at least ten of the fifteen surveys are included in the study.

n.a. Not available.

a. Included in 1968 data.

b. Number of beds in year of adoption or, if that was not available, number of beds the year before or after adoption.

combined and a hospital was considered to have adopted intensive care in the first year in which it reported either type of unit.[19]

Table 3-3 shows the distribution of the 1,705 hospitals by the year in which the hospital introduced intensive care. The distribution corresponds closely to the pattern shown in figure 3-1, which charts the national trends for private nonprofit hospitals: adoption was rapid during the 1960s and

19. The criteria for assigning the year of adoption were actually more complicated, to allow for inaccuracies and nonresponses, and included the rule that a hospital was considered to have adopted intensive care in the first of *two consecutive* years in which it reported either type of unit. Other criteria insured that this represented the start of a period in which the hospital consistently reported having intensive care.

tapered off in the 1970s as it approached the saturation point. The table starts with the year 1962 because it was impossible to distinguish hospitals that adopted in 1961, the first year for which information was available, from those that had had units for several years and were simply reporting the fact again. There is also a gap in 1966 and 1967 because the AHA omitted intensive care, along with a number of other facilities, from the survey in those years; as a result, the number of hospitals shown as introducing intensive care in 1968 is overstated because it includes hospitals that had actually established units a year or two earlier but did not get a chance to report the event until 1968. The table also shows the breakdown of the hospitals by size.

The purpose of the statistical analysis is to try to identify the reasons some hospitals adopted intensive care more quickly than others. The two regressions in table 3-4 are the distillation of this analysis and show the differences—expressed in years and fractions of years—associated with the characteristics of hospitals and their markets discussed in chapter 2. As explained in that chapter, the data measuring third party payment are subject to a number of serious problems and so the first equation gives the results when third party payment is omitted, the second the results when it is included.

The characteristics that may help to explain why certain kinds of hospitals adopted intensive care more or less quickly are listed down the left-hand side of the table. For each, the sample of hospitals is divided into two or more classes: there are those that are affiliated with a medical school and those that are not; those that offer general medical and surgical services and those that are more specialized; those with fewer than 100 beds, with 100 through 199 beds, with 200 through 299 beds, and with 300 beds or more; and so on. The table shows the increase or decrease in the number of years until intensive care was adopted associated with each particular class.[20]

One class of each characteristic, or factor, is labeled the reference class and has no number beside it. This class serves as the basis of comparison for the other classes of the same factor. To illustrate, hospitals with 100 through 199 beds adopted intensive care an estimated 1.32 years sooner, on average, than did hospitals with fewer than 100 beds, the reference

20. The number in parentheses next to this estimate is its *t*-statistic. Where the *t*-statistic shows that the estimate is different from zero at the 90 or 95 percent levels of confidence, this is indicated by the asterisks, which are defined more precisely in the footnotes to the table.

Table 3-4. The Year in Which Intensive Care Was Adopted by a Hospital, 1961–75: Differences Associated with Selected Characteristics of the Hospital and Its Market[a]

	Year	
Characteristic	*Regression excluding third party payment*	*Regression including third party payment*
Year for hospitals with all the reference characteristics[b]	1969.72 (77.7)**	1969.81 (73.8)**
	Differences associated with size, control, and service	
Beds[c]		
Under 100	Reference class	Reference class
100–199	−1.32 (7.1)**	−1.32 (7.1)**
200–299	−2.83 (12.3)**	−2.84 (12.3)**
300 and over	−3.25 (12.2)**	−3.26 (12.2)**
Control		
Private nonprofit	Reference class	Reference class
State and local government	+0.83 (4.2)**	+0.83 (4.2)**
Private, profit	+0.77 (3.3)**	+0.80 (3.3)**
Service		
General	Reference class	Reference class
Specialized	+1.92 (4.3)**	+1.94 (4.3)**
	Differences associated with teaching and research	
Medical school affiliation		
Yes	−0.55 (2.1)**	−0.55 (2.1)**
No	Reference class	Reference class
Residents per 100 beds[c]		
0	Reference class	Reference class
1–9	−0.71 (3.6)**	−0.71 (3.5)**
10–19	−0.91 (2.5)**	−0.93 (2.6)**
20 and over	−0.33 (0.6)	−0.36 (0.7)
Research grants to hospitals, dollars per bed		
0	Reference class	Reference class
1–99	+0.21 (0.9)	+0.18 (0.7)
100–999	−0.30 (1.1)	−0.32 (1.1)
1,000 and over	−0.36 (1.1)	−0.44 (1.3)
	Differences associated with patient care	
Doctors per 1,000 beds		
Under 175	+0.37 (1.5)	+0.36 (1.4)
175–249	Reference class	Reference class
250 and over	−0.12 (0.6)	−0.09 (0.4)
Deaths from heart disease per 1,000 beds		
Under 350	−0.56 (1.8)*	−0.53 (1.7)*
350–449	−0.35 (1.4)	−0.31 (1.2)
450–549	−0.10 (0.4)	−0.08 (0.3)
550–649	Reference class	Reference class
650 and over	+0.15 (0.6)	+0.12 (0.5)

Table 3-4 (*continued*)

Characteristic	Year	
	Regression excluding third party payment	*Regression including third party payment*
Differences associated with patient care (continued)		
Deaths from motor vehicle accidents per 1,000 beds		
Under 30	+0.02 (0.1)	+0.03 (0.1)
30–44	Reference class	Reference class
45–59	+0.09 (0.4)	+0.10 (0.5)
60 and over	−0.27 (1.0)	−0.23 (0.9)
Percent of population white		
Under 85	+0.56 (3.2)**	+0.56 (3.0)**
85–94	Reference class	Reference class
95 and over		0.12 (0.6)		0.06 (0.3)
Differences associated with market structure		
Percent of beds in four largest hospitals		
Under 50	Reference class	Reference class
50–79	+0.06 (0.3)	+0.09 (0.4)
80–100	+0.23 (0.8)	+0.25 (0.8)
Market with fewer than four hospitals	+0.12 (0.3)	+0.14 (0.4)
Percent growth in population, 1960–70		
Under 15	Reference class	Reference class
15–24	−0.40 (1.9)*	−0.37 (1.7)*
25 and over	−0.56 (2.4)**	−0.50 (2.1)**
Percent of hospitals with intensive care in 1961		
0	−0.25 (1.0)	−0.18 (0.7)
1–14	−0.05 (0.2)	+0.04 (0.2)
15–29	Reference class	Reference class
30 and over	−0.58 (2.5)**	−0.47 (1.9)*
Differences associated with third party payment		
Percent of population with hospital insurance, 1963		
Under 65	...	−0.17 (0.4)
65–74	...	−0.06 (0.2)
75–84	...	−0.12 (0.4)
85 and over	...	Reference class
Percent growth in hospital insurance, 1961–71		
Under 10	...	−0.35 (1.0)
10–19	...	Reference class
20–29	...	−0.28 (1.0)
30 and over	...	−0.17 (0.6)
Differences associated with regulation		
Effective year, certificate-of-need law		
1965–69	+0.20 (0.7)	+0.25 (0.7)
1970–73	−0.15 (0.9)	−0.04 (0.2)
1974–75 or no law	Reference class	Reference class

Table 3-4 (*continued*)

	Year	
Characteristic	*Regression excluding third party payment*	*Regression including third party payment*
Summary statistic		
Number of observations	1,705	1,705
R^2	0.267	0.268
Corrected R^2	0.252	0.251
F and degrees of freedom [numerator, denominator]	17.87 [34, 1670]	15.21 [40, 1664]

Sources: See chapter 2 for discussion of the basic data.

*The difference is statistically significant at the 90 percent level of confidence or better, but less than the 95 percent level.

** The difference is statistically significant at the 95 percent level of confidence or better.

a. The numbers in parentheses are *t*-statistics.

b. This is the constant term of the regression and shows the estimated year of adoption for hospitals having all the reference characteristics. (See text for explanation of the notion of a reference class.) The values of the dependent variable used in the regressions ranged from 22 (for 1962) to 35 (for 1975), but the constant is expressed here in terms of the corresponding calendar year to make its interpretation more obvious. The *t*-statistic in this case applies not to the number shown but to the difference between that number and 1940 (to 1969.72 − 1940 = 29.72 in column 1, for example).

c. In the year intensive care was adopted, or, if not available, the year before or after.

class. Similarly, each of the other estimates should be read as the difference in the speed of adoption between hospitals in that class and hospitals in the reference class.[21]

21. Following the standard statistical technique, binary variables were defined for each class of an explanatory factor except the reference class. These variables are assigned the value 1 for a hospital in the particular class and 0 for all other hospitals. Each hospital is in only one class. Hospitals in the reference class are also uniquely defined since they are the only observations assigned values of 0 for all of the variables.

Whenever a single explanatory factor—number of beds, for example—is represented by several binary variables, there ought, strictly speaking, to be a test of the significance of the group of binaries taken as a whole. The appropriate test is the *F*-ratio for the group (Emanuel Melichar, "Least-Squares Analysis of Economic Survey Data," American Statistical Association, *Proceedings of the Business and Economic Statistics Section, 1965* [Washington, D.C.: ASA], pp. 373–85). However, in an earlier study using the same statistical techniques (Louise B. Russell and Carol S. Burke, *Determinants of Infant and Child Mortality: An Econometric Analysis of Survey Data for San Juan, Argentina,* prepared for the Agency for International Development [National Planning Association, February 1975]), it was discovered that, whenever at least one of the *t*-statistics for a group of binaries was significant, the *F*-ratio was significant, and when none of them was, the *F* was not significant. Thus nothing appeared to be gained, and to save time and expense, the group *F*s were not calculated in this study. The discussion in the text is based on the generalization that whenever at least one binary is statistically significant, the group is significant.

Finally, it should be noted that the *t*-statistic for each estimate shows only whether the difference between the particular class and the reference class is sta-

The ultimate point of reference is the year shown at the top of the table. This is an estimate of the year in which hospitals with *all* the characteristics represented by the reference classes—fewer than 100 beds, private nonprofit control, general service, no medical school affiliation, no residents, and so on—adopted intensive care. The estimated year for these hospitals is late 1969 (1969.72 in column 1, 1969.81 in column 2). An estimate of the year for hospitals with any other combination of characteristics can be derived by starting with this base year and adding or subtracting the differences associated with the particular characteristics chosen. For example, for a hospital with all the reference characteristics except that it has 350 beds and a small residency program, the estimate—based on the regression in the first column of the table—is 1965.76 (1969.72 − 3.25   0.71).

It is clear from the results shown in the table that the size of the hospital—which is a first approximation to the scale of all its activities—is an important determinant of the speed with which it adopted intensive care. Hospitals with 100 through 199 beds adopted it in some form about 1.3 years earlier than hospitals with fewer than 100 beds, those with 200 through 299 beds about 2.8 years earlier, and those with 300 or more beds a little earlier still, by about 3.3 years. This is consistent both with the national trends graphed in figure 3-1 and with the fact that larger hospitals have correspondingly more patients, doctors, and residents to benefit from the new technology.

Even after size is taken into account, private nonprofit hospitals were faster off the mark. State and local government hospitals and profit hospitals lagged nearly a year behind (more precisely, about 0.8 of a year in both cases). Specialized hospitals were slower than general hospitals, by almost two years, to establish intensive care units.

Teaching responsibilities influenced the speed of adoption, but research grants did not. Hospitals affiliated with medical schools established units about six months earlier (0.55 of a year), on average, than those without

---

tistically significant. The differences between any other combination of two classes may also be significant. The reader can calculate an approximate t-statistic to discover whether this is the case in any particular instance by using the formula $\sqrt{\sigma_1^2 + \sigma_2^2}$, where σ_1^2 and σ_2^2 are the variances associated with the estimates for the two classes of interest. These variances are not shown in the tables, but can be derived by dividing each estimate by its own t-statistic, shown in parentheses beside it, and squaring the result. The approximate t-statistic for the difference between the two estimates is then the ratio of that difference to the term calculated from the formula.

such an affiliation. Residency programs speeded the process even more—by almost a year. The results for residents are probably best interpreted as meaning that hospitals with a program differed from those without one, but that the size of the program was not very important. The estimates for one through nine residents and ten through nineteen residents per 100 beds are not significantly different from each other, and the number of hospitals in the highest class—twenty or more residents—is so small that this estimate is probably not very reliable. From this point of view, it might have been better to combine the two highest classes, but this was not done because it seemed best to maintain comparability between the classes defined for this analysis and those defined for the analysis of the distribution of intensive care beds.

Few clear-cut relationships appear among the factors related to the care of patients. The estimates show some tendency for intensive care to be adopted more slowly where there are fewer doctors and more quickly where doctors are abundant, but none of the differences are significant at even the 90 percent level. Deaths from motor vehicle accidents show no important connection with the adoption of intensive care, and while deaths from heart disease are related, the relationship is an unexpected one—intensive care was introduced more quickly by hospitals in areas with the fewest deaths. This pattern appears again in the next section and in the analysis of open-heart surgery in chapter 5. The possibility that the technology has produced a measurable reduction in total deaths can be ruled out in the case of open-heart surgery, since the data on deaths are for a period when open-heart procedures were still uncommon. And given that the bulk of the deaths from heart attack occur before the patient reaches a hospital, and that studies of the effects of intensive care on those who do get to the hospital have gotten mixed results (see the last section of this chapter), it seems unlikely that the relationship is one of causality in this case, either. But here the interpretation cannot be ruled out completely. Finally, adoption proceeded somewhat more slowly in areas with large nonwhite populations.

The speed with which hospitals established intensive care units is not related to market concentration (as measured by the percent of beds controlled by the four largest hospitals), but market growth is important. In areas where the population grew by 15 to 24 percent between 1960 and 1970, hospitals adopted intensive care several months faster than hospitals in areas where the growth was less, and where the growth exceeded 25 percent, adoption was faster still, by about half a year.

Reflecting the impetus for diffusion provided by example, hospitals that had not yet introduced intensive care by 1961, but that were located in markets where 30 percent or more of the hospitals had, subsequently adopted the technology about six months sooner than other hospitals. This factor may represent both the specific competitive pressures for this technology and the local availability of information about it. The result is consistent with studies of diffusion in other industries, which have found that the higher the proportion of firms that have already adopted an innovation, the faster the remaining firms adopt it.[22]

Two of the measures of third party payment—the percent of the population with hospital insurance and the growth in that percent—show no effect on the speed of adoption. It is impossible to know for certain whether these results reflect the reality for this particular technology or the limitations of the data, but the limitations are sufficiently severe (see chapter 2) that the latter explanation is more likely. In this analysis, it was difficult to make use of the better-quality data on the percent of hospital costs paid by Medicare because of the strong definitional relation between Medicare and the speed of diffusion: the hospitals that introduced intensive care early, before Medicare started in mid-1966, could not be influenced by it. A crude method of including these data, which involved splitting the constant term into two parts (1966 or before, and after 1966), was tested and the result was a lot of collinearity and no evidence that Medicare influenced the speed of diffusion among the late adopters.[23]

The same difficulty got in the way of testing the effects of the regional medical program (RMP) and comprehensive health planning (CHP) program—neither of which existed before the late 1960s—on the diffusion of intensive care. The method used with the Medicare data was also tried for RMP and no significant effect appeared.

A similar problem, but less debilitating, existed for certificate-of-need laws, which were introduced by the states over a number of years beginning in 1965. The obvious approach—to distinguish between hospitals adopting intensive care before a certificate-of-need law was passed and

22. Edwin Mansfield, *Industrial Research and Technological Innovation: An Econometric Analysis* (Norton, 1968), chap. 7.
23. An analysis of national trends by size of hospital, reported elsewhere, showed that the speed of diffusion among hospitals with fewer than 100 beds increased after Medicare began, but that larger hospitals were unaffected. Louise B. Russell, "The Diffusion of Hospital Technologies: Some Econometric Evidence," *Journal of Human Resources,* vol. 12 (Fall 1977), pp. 482–502.

those adopting after—was not possible because only late adopters were subject to the law, and the definitional relationship overwhelms any behavioral effects. But in the states with earlier laws a larger proportion of *all* adopters were subject to them, and it is thus reasonable to define classes—according to the effective year of the law—which include all hospitals in the state, even if they introduced intensive care before the law.[24] The only shortcoming of this approach is that the resulting estimates are averages over groups that include hospitals on which certificate-of-need clearly had no effect. As the table shows, these estimates do not indicate that the average effect was significant.

The reader will be heartened to know that the difficulties of testing the Medicare and regulatory data are limited to the analyses of the speed of diffusion here and in chapter 4 (and in chapter 4, respiratory therapy is the exception to the rule, because the data for that technology do not begin until 1968). They do not apply to the analyses in the next section and in chapter 5, and it is thus possible to learn some interesting things about these programs in the course of the study.

The Statistical Analysis: The Distribution of Intensive Care Beds among Hospitals, 1975

The number of beds devoted to intensive care by different types of hospitals varies widely—in large part, of course, because of differences in size: a hospital with only 100 beds, and the patient load that goes with it, will not need as many beds in intensive care as will a hospital with 400 beds. But even when the number of intensive care beds is expressed as a percentage of the total number of beds in the hospital, considerable variation remains. Among the 2,772 hospitals selected from the 1975 survey, this percentage ranges from zero to 40 percent around an average of 5 percent.[25] Table 3-5 shows the complete distribution.

24. The proportion of hospitals subject to a certificate-of-need law (defined as those that reported introducing intensive care at least one year after the law went into effect) was 53 percent for hospitals in states with laws effective between 1965 and 1969, 10 percent for hospitals in states with laws between 1970 and 1973, and less than 1 percent for the reference class—a law in either 1974 or 1975, or no law.

25. A few of the zeroes may be hospitals that did not respond to the question about intensive care beds. The two observations with values of 40 percent are not so obviously due to mistakes in the data as one might think at first. Both are small children's hospitals in large cities (Boston and San Francisco) and it is quite plausible that they are so highly specialized as to have that many beds in intensive care. The third highest observation is 27 percent. That hospital and the remaining eleven with values of 20 percent or more are also located in large cities.

Table 3-5. Distributions of Study Hospitals by Percent of Beds in Intensive Care and Coronary Care Units, Total and by Size of Hospital, 1975

Percent of beds in intensive care and coronary care units	All study hospitals		Hospitals by number of beds			
	Number	Percent	Under 100	100–199	200–299	300 and over
None	348	12.6	290	52	3	3
Under 2.0	44	1.6	0	13	10	21
2.0–2.9	219	7.9	14	62	46	97
3.0–3.9	369	13.3	25	87	88	169
4.0–4.9	509	18.4	64	125	101	219
5.0–5.9	420	15.2	67	128	99	126
6.0–6.9	280	10.1	63	85	58	74
7.0–7.9	198	7.1	50	62	42	44
8.0–8.9	135	4.9	48	33	26	28
9.0–9.9	72	2.6	16	29	10	17
10 and over	178	6.4	62	64	23	29
Total	2,772	100.0	699	740	506	827
Percent of total	...	...	25.2	26.7	18.3	29.8

Source: AHA's 1975 survey of hospitals.

This section tries to explain the differences among hospitals in the percentage of beds they allocate to intensive care. The results of the analysis are set out in table 3-6, which shows two regressions, one without and one with the third party payment data.

This time, the numbers in the table are estimates of the differences in the percentage of beds in intensive care (the differences are expressed as percents) associated with the particular characteristic of the hospital or its market. The base percent, listed at the top of the table, is the percentage for hospitals having all the reference-class characteristics—fewer than 100 beds, private nonprofit control, general service, no medical school affiliation, and so on. In both regressions this base estimate is a bit more than 3 percent: 3.38 percent when third party payment is omitted, 3.08 percent when it is included. An estimate for any other type of hospital can be derived by starting with the base percent and adding or subtracting the differences associated with its particular characteristics.[26]

The differences associated with the total number of beds in the hospital show that the relationship between intensive care beds and total beds is not strictly proportional. Instead, while the percentage of beds in intensive care is consistently higher for hospitals with more than 100 beds than for

26. To avoid awkwardness, the shorthand term "intensive care beds" is used in the text to mean "the percent of total beds allocated to intensive care."

Table 3-6. Percent of Beds Committed to Intensive Care by a Hospital, 1975: Differences Associated with Selected Characteristics of the Hospital and Its Market[a]

	Percent of beds in intensive care	
Characteristic	Regression excluding third party payment	Regression including third party payment
Percent for hospitals with all the reference characteristics[b]	3.38 (9.4)**	3.08 (7.5)**
	Differences associated with size, control, and service	
Beds		
Under 100	Reference class	Reference class
100–199	+1.37 (7.8)**	+1.39 (7.9)**
200–299	+1.16 (5.7)**	+1.16 (5.7)**
300 and over	+0.60 (2.8)**	+0.63 (2.9)**
Control		
Private nonprofit	Reference class	Reference class
State and local government	−0.56 (3.1)**	−0.59 (3.3)**
Private, profit	−0.31 (1.6)	−0.39 (1.9)*
Service		
General	Reference class	Reference class
Specialized	−1.01 (3.4)**	−1.01 (3.4)**
	Differences associated with teaching and research	
Medical school affiliation		
Yes	+0.69 (3.1)**	+0.71 (3.2)**
No	Reference class	Reference class
Residents per 100 beds		
0	Reference class	Reference class
1–9	−0.32 (1.7)*	−0.32 (1.7)*
10–19	−0.48 (1.6)	−0.47 (1.6)
20 and over	+0.74 (2.1)**	+0.76 (2.2)**
Research grants to hospitals, dollars per bed		
0	Reference class	Reference class
1–99	−0.18 (0.8)	−0.13 (0.6)
100–999	+0.02 (0.1)	+0.19 (0.7)
1,000 and over	+0.67 (2.2)**	+1.02 (3.2)**
	Differences associated with patient care	
Doctors per 1,000 beds		
Under 175	−0.46 (2.1)**	−0.54 (2.3)**
175–249	Reference class	Reference class
250 and over	+0.15 (0.8)	−0.05 (0.2)
Deaths from heart disease per 1,000 beds		
Under 350	+0.29 (1.1)	+0.50 (1.7)*
350–449	+0.18 (0.8)	+0.30 (1.3)
450–549	+0.06 (0.3)	+0.09 (0.4)
550–649	Reference class	Reference class
650 and over	+0.11 (0.5)	+0.03 (0.1)

Table 3-6 (*continued*)

	Percent of beds in intensive care	
Characteristic	*Regression excluding third party payment*	*Regression including third party payment*
Differences associated with patient care (*continued*)		
Deaths from motor vehicle accidents per 1,000 beds		
Under 30	−0.06 (0.3)	+0.06 (0.3)
30–44	Reference class	Reference class
45–59	+0.06 (0.3)	+0.08 (0.4)
60 and over	+0.43 (1.8)*	+0.57 (2.3)**
Percent of population white		
Under 85	−0.36 (2.2)**	−0.33 (1.8)*
85–94	Reference class	Reference class
95 and over	+0.27 (1.4)	+0.30 (1.4)
Differences associated with market structure		
Percent of beds in four largest hospitals		
Under 50	Reference class	Reference class
50–79	+0.16 (0.7)	+0.15 (0.7)
80–100	−0.20 (0.8)	−0.27 (1.1)
Market with fewer than four hospitals	+0.18 (0.5)	+0.07 (0.2)
Percent growth in population, 1960–70		
Under 15	Reference class	Reference class
15–24	+0.60 (3.1)**	+0.56 (2.8)**
25 and over	+1.07 (4.7)**	+0.90 (3.6)**
Percent of beds committed to intensive care in other hospitals		
Under 2	−0.45 (2.1)**	−0.36 (1.6)*
2–5	Reference class	Reference class
6 and over	+0.41 (2.3)**	+0.26 (1.3)
Differences associated with third party payment		
Percent of population with hospital insurance, 1963		
Under 65	...	+0.43 (1.1)
65–74	...	+0.28 (0.9)
75–84	...	+0.11 (0.4)
85 and over	...	Reference class
Percent growth in hospital insurance, 1961–71		
Under 10	...	+0.52 (1.5)
10–19	...	Reference class
20–29	...	+0.33 (1.3)
30 and over	...	+0.31 (1.1)
Percent of costs paid by Medicare		
Under 15	...	−0.14 (0.4)
15–19	...	−0.41 (2.1)**
20–24	...	Reference class
25–29	...	+0.32 (1.4)
30 and over	...	+0.37 (1.0)

Table 3-6 (*continued*)

	Percent of beds in intensive care	
Characteristic	*Regression excluding third party payment*	*Regression including third party payment*
	Differences associated with regulation	
Effective year, certificate-of-need law		
1965–69	−0.68 (2.4)**	−0.87 (2.5)**
1970–73	+0.13 (0.8)	−0.07 (0.4)
1974–75 or no law	Reference class	Reference class
Regional medical program dollars per hospital		
Under 100,000	Reference class	Reference class
100,000 and over	+0.42 (2.9)**	+0.42 (2.5)**
Area comprehensive health planning dollars per hospital		
0	+0.25 (1.0)	+0.16 (0.6)
1–4,999	−0.07 (0.3)	+0.02 (0.1)
5,000–14,999	Reference class	Reference class
15,000 and over	+0.14 (0.7)	+0.17 (0.9)
Summary statistic		
Number of observations	2,772	2,772
R^2	0.111	0.116
Corrected R^2	0.099	0.101
F and degrees of freedom [numerator, denominator]	9.19 [37, 2734]	7.62 [47, 2724]

Sources: See chapter 2 for discussion of the basic data.
* The difference is statistically significant at the 90 percent level of confidence or better, but less than the 95 percent level.
** The difference is statistically significant at the 95 percent level of confidence or better.
a. The numbers in parentheses are *t*-statistics.
b. This is the constant term of the regression and shows the percentage of beds committed to intensive care in hospitals having all the reference characteristics. (See text for explanation of the notion of a reference class.)

hospitals with fewer, the difference declines as the number of beds increases—from +1.4 percent for hospitals of 100 through 199 beds to +1.2 percent for those with 200 through 299 beds and +0.6 percent for larger hospitals. For hospitals that differ from the reference class only in size, these estimates correspond to total percentages of, from the first column, 4.75 (3.38 + 1.37), 4.54 (3.38 + 1.16), and 3.98 (3.38 + 0.60), respectively.

This pattern is consistent with the idea that certain sizes and configurations of units are viewed as desirable, regardless of the size of the hospital, and that as soon as a hospital is within hailing distance of being able to make use of such units, it tries to introduce them. For example, although a unit of four beds is considered to be economically feasible, a minimum of eight beds is considered necessary for real efficiency, and some value is attached to having a separate unit for coronary patients. A mixed ICU of eight beds and a separate CCU of four or more would clearly overwhelm a hospital of only fifty beds; they would be feasible, but well above the base percent, for a hospital of 200 beds. Larger hospitals would want to add other types of units or more beds to accommodate the specialized care they give, so that the percentage difference might decline but it would not disappear.

Just as they adopted intensive care later, state and local hospitals and hospitals operated for profit have committed relatively fewer beds to it than nonprofit hospitals; the difference is more than half a percent for state and local hospitals, somewhat smaller for profit hospitals. Similarly, the substantial delay in the adoption of intensive care units by specialized hospitals is matched by a lower percentage of beds allocated to them; the estimate of −1.0 percent is larger than either of the differences associated with control, or, for that matter, than most of the differences in the table.[27]

Medical school affiliation raises the level of intensive care beds by about 0.7 percent, but residency programs have a mixed effect. Although hospitals with small or medium-sized programs adopted intensive care earlier, they allocate somewhat fewer beds to it than hospitals without programs; the differences are small—about one bed less for a 300-bed hospital, two less for a 600-bed hospital. On the other hand, hospitals with large residency programs have significantly more beds in intensive care. Similarly, hospitals with large research programs have more intensive care beds—their percentage averages 0.67 to 1.02 points higher—than those with no research, but more modest research programs have no effect.

Hospitals in areas with few doctors relative to the number of hospital beds have fewer intensive care beds, in line with the hypothesis that where there are fewer doctors there is less pressure to adopt or, in this case, expand new technologies. The relationship does not extend beyond the lowest class: hospitals in areas with the greatest abundance of doctors, 250 or more per 1,000 beds, are not noticeably different from those

27. It frequently happens in this chapter that a factor that is associated with a slower speed of adoption is also associated with a lower percentage of beds in intensive care. Since the rapid growth of intensive care beds in recent years indicates that the diffusion process is not complete, it may be that the later adopters were further from their ultimate level of beds in 1975 and that if and when they reach that level some of the differences between them and the hospitals that adopted earlier will diminish or even disappear.

in areas with between 175 and 249 doctors. Experimentation produced no evidence that the specialty distribution influenced the level of beds, and thus these data were not included in the regressions in table 3-6.

Where the number of deaths from motor vehicle accidents is especially high (sixty or more per 1,000 beds), hospitals devote more of their beds to intensive care. Deaths from heart disease, however, have an effect that is consistent with the curious pattern that showed up in the last section, but weaker: hospitals in areas with fewer deaths have a slightly higher percentage of beds in intensive care than do those in areas where there are more deaths.[28] As for the last of the patient care characteristics shown in the table, hospitals in areas with a large proportion of nonwhites allocate fewer beds to intensive care.

The degree of concentration in the market has no effect on intensive care beds—as it had no effect on the speed of diffusion—but hospitals in faster growing markets have significantly more beds in ICUs than do hospitals in the slowest growing markets. Where the growth in population from 1960 to 1970 fell between 15 and 25 percent, the difference is about 0.6 percent. Where it exceeded 25 percent, the difference is 1 full percentage point. And in spite of the fact that competition as measured by concentration has no effect, hospitals once again appear to be influenced by the examples of those around them. They have fewer beds in intensive care when the hospitals around them have fewer, and more beds when the hospitals around them have more.

Neither the percentage of the population with hospital insurance nor the growth in that percentage demonstrates any effect on intensive care beds; again, this may reflect the limitations of the data. In this analysis it was also possible to test the Medicare data. With the exception of the lowest class—less than 15 percent of hospital costs paid by Medicare— these data show a smooth and statistically significant relationship with intensive care beds: where Medicare payments are higher, the percentage of beds in intensive care is higher.[29] The difference between hospitals in SMSAs in which Medicare paid 15 through 19 percent of costs and those in SMSAs in which it paid 20 through 24 percent (the reference class) is statistically significant. The differences between the 15 through 19 percent class and the classes above 25 percent are even stronger (see note 21),

28. In the regression excluding third party payment, none of the differences is statistically significant at even the 90 percent level.

29. The percentage of the population sixty-five years old or older did not show any relationship to intensive care beds and was not included in the regressions in table 3-6.

although these classes are not significantly different at the 90 percent level from the closer reference class.

Given the weaknesses of the data on third party payment, the results of greatest interest are probably those for the three programs grouped under regulation—certificate-of-need laws, the regional medical program, and the comprehensive health planning program—all of which could be properly tested in this analysis. Comprehensive health planning programs have no effect on the percentage of intensive care beds. But regional medical programs spending $100,000 or more raised the percentage of intensive care beds in their areas about 0.4 percent above the level in areas spending less than $100,000. This is entirely consistent with the history of the program, briefly sketched in chapter 2. The regional programs focused on intensive care right from the start and, as the results show, were successful in promoting it.

The early certificate-of-need laws have also had an important effect, but in the direction of reducing the percentage of beds allocated to intensive care. As noted in chapter 2, hospitals in New York dominate this group, so that it is probably more accurate to say that the New York review program has had a significant effect. The estimated reduction is on the order of 0.7 to 0.9 percent. Application of the formula developed earlier in this chapter indicates (assuming hospitals did not offset this restraint by investing in some other direction, which is the crucial question) that an effect of this size translates into a cost per hospital day approximately 1.5 percent lower than would have been true in the absence of certificate-of-need. More recent laws have yet to make a difference in intensive care, whether from lack of opportunity or because the reviewers in these states do not perceive intensive care as overexpanded.

The results of the analyses of intensive care are interesting in their own right, the more so because they apply to a technology central to the modern hospital. But the patterns that are confirmed by repetition across several technologies have the greatest importance for policy, and for this reason, further summary and discussion of the results presented in the last two sections will be left to chapter 7, when conclusions can be drawn based on the entire study.

The Benefits of Intensive Care

Intensive care is expensive, it is widespread, and it is growing. What are we getting for the money? The answer to this question has to be built piece by piece, because patients with different conditions receive intensive care and the benefits may not be the same for all of them, and because there are several kinds of potential benefit, although the saving of lives is considered the most important. This discussion is limited to the effects of intensive care that benefit the patient directly; others can argue the case for its contribution to medical teaching and research.

Perhaps the best way to begin is to present a sampling of results from studies of several different but fairly common conditions. Stroke, for example, is one of the major causes of death, and some hospitals have special intensive care units for it. One article on the subject noted that three earlier studies of individual stroke units had produced two findings of no effect and one finding of a dramatic reduction in mortality.[30] The authors' own study compared 100 stroke patients admitted to the stroke unit in their hospital to eighty-one stroke patients treated in the neurology ward. The results were potentially biased because the patients admitted to the stroke unit tended to be more seriously ill. After omitting the early deaths from both groups to correct for this bias, the authors concluded that the mortality rates were about the same—that there was no advantage to intensive care.

A considerably more ambitious study was published at about the same time.[31] The study followed six hospitals for a period before and after the introduction of stroke units in three of them. This design made it possible for the investigators to observe the differences between the two groups of hospitals before any had stroke units and the changes that occurred after the units were introduced and thus gave the investigators confidence that the results they attributed to the stroke units were actually due to the units and not to other differences between the two groups of hospitals. But, after making further corrections for the condition of the patients at the time they were brought to the hospital, the authors concluded that the mortality rate was no better in the hospitals with stroke units than in those without. They did find two more modest advantages: patients admitted to the hospitals with stroke units developed fewer complications; and more of them improved over the course of their hospital stay in their ability to care for themselves.[32]

30. Samuel E. Pitner and Cornelius J. Mance, "An Evaluation of Stroke Intensive Care: Results in a Municipal Hospital," Stroke, vol. 4 (September–October 1973), pp. 737–41.

31. William E. Drake, Jr., and others, "Acute Stroke Management and Patient Outcome: The Value of Neurovascular Care Units (NCU)," Stroke, vol. 4 (November–December 1973), pp. 933–45.

32. The comparisons were made between all stroke patients admitted to the

Several studies of intensive care have been carried out by Paul F. Griner and his colleagues in Rochester, New York. In one, Griner examined the experience of patients with acute pulmonary edema (accumulation of fluid in the lungs) in the year before and the year after the opening of an intensive care unit in the study hospital; he found no difference in mortality between the two years, although the more seriously ill patients were admitted to the ICU in the later years.[33] Kenneth W. Piper and Paul Griner investigated the effect of intensive care on people who had tried to commit suicide by taking an overdose of drugs.[34] Here, too, they found no difference in mortality rates. They did find that patients who received intensive care had fewer complications and shorter hospital stays, but neither difference was statistically significant, and the shorter stays were attributed to better discharge planning in the ICU rather than better care.

A great many studies, of varying quality, have been done of intensive care for heart attacks (myocardial infarction).[35] Some of them do show a reduction in the mortality rate with intensive care, but at least an equal number do not. One carefully designed British study—it may be the only study of myocardial infarction ever to assign patients randomly to different types of care—examined an alternative seldom mentioned in the United States: *home* care.[36] The study found that, overall, there was no difference in mortality between heart-attack patients given intensive care and those treated at home. When the results were examined in detail, they showed that one group of patients—those over sixty years old who did not have low blood pressure immediately following the attack—actually did significantly better at home.

As this quick review suggests, it is difficult to design a convincing test of intensive care's effectiveness. It is obviously necessary to control for

---

hospitals with units and all those admitted to the control hospitals, although some of the patients in the former group were treated on the wards.

33. Griner, "Treatment of Acute Pulmonary Edema."

34. Kenneth W. Piper and Paul F. Griner, "Suicide Attempts with Drug Overdose: Outcomes of Intensive vs Conventional Floor Care," *Archives of Internal Medicine,* vol. 134 (October 1974), pp. 703–06.

35. See, for example, the review and study by K. Astvad and others, "Mortality from Acute Myocardial Infarction Before and After Establishment of a Coronary Care Unit," *British Medical Journal,* vol. 1 (March 23, 1974), pp. 567–69.

36. H. G. Mather and others, "Myocardial Infarction: A Comparison between Home and Hospital Care for Patients," *British Medical Journal,* vol. 1 (April 17, 1976), pp. 925–29.

differences among patients, and, when the test compares hospitals, for differences among hospitals, but it is not an easy matter to do so. Careful definitions have to be established at the beginning—for example, the symptoms and laboratory tests that are sufficient to establish whether a suspected myocardial infarction or stroke really is one—so that the groups compared are truly comparable. Without such controls and definitions, the results may be swamped by the variability among hospitals, among patients, and even among investigators.

The practical difficulties can be quite complex. How, for example, if the comparison is between groups of patients in the same hospital, can one be certain that the care given ward patients has not been changed by the introduction of the special unit into the hospital, so that the entire medical and nursing staff pays more attention to certain signs and symptoms? If this is the case, the true difference between ward care and intensive care will be understated.[37]

If the comparison is the before-and-after type, comparing an earlier and a later year, the problem is to control for major changes in the types of patients admitted to the CCU and for changes in treatment other than those associated with the CCU itself. For example, Geoffrey Rose presents three facts about Britain: the in-hospital mortality rate from acute coronary heart disease has declined; the number of patients with acute coronary heart disease admitted to hospitals has increased; the mortality rate from coronary heart disease in the population as a whole has remained the same.[38] (All three items are standardized by age.) He concludes that the decline in hospital mortality has not been due to intensive care but to the increasing hospitalization of mild cases—cases in which the patient is less likely to die, no matter what treatment is given—as the hospital has become the accepted place of treatment for heart disease. A corresponding trend has been observed in the United States, where the proportion of patients in CCUs who actually have myocardial infarctions has declined over the years, and more and more patients with other coronary conditions—most of which have a much lower fatality rate—have been admitted.[39]

37. Killip and Kimball, "A Survey of the Coronary Care Unit."
38. Geoffrey Rose, "The Contribution of Intensive Coronary Care," *British Journal of Preventive and Social Medicine,* vol. 29 (September 1975), pp. 147–50.
39. "An Analysis of Cardiac Care Unit Experiences: The Virginia Regional Medical Program's Cardiac Unit Study Group," *Virginia Medical Monthly,* vol. 102 (March 1975), pp. 205–13.

How can one be certain that the place of treatment does not affect the course of the illness in ways that bias the results? For example, some studies look at the number of cardiac arrests that occur and compare the success of each place of treatment in resuscitating these patients. Coronary care units unquestionably do better at this, and yet the mortality rate of patients cared for at home is just as good. This has led several observers to wonder, quite seriously, whether the stress of being in the hospital might not *cause* cardiac arrest in some patients.[40]

Obviously, it is no easy matter to design a study that avoids all the problems people have thought of, let alone those they will think of after the study is done. This is part of the reason intensive care has continued its exuberant growth in the face of the rather lackluster evidence about its effects. The rest of the reason has to do with the enthusiasm and faith that are invested in new medical technologies. Intensive care is a very appealing technology. It sounds like it ought to work. It satisfies people's need to do something impressive in a crisis. It is much more convenient than caring for a patient at home, in cases where that is a possibility, and lets the doctor and the patient share responsibility for the outcome with other people. It is a great environment for teaching and research. Altogether, it is not surprising that faith plays a large part in maintaining the popularity of intensive care.

The strength of that faith is well illustrated by two specific examples. Both have to do with doctors, but the faith is shared by much of the public as well. In the first example, a study that examined the effect of a CCU on mortality from myocardial infarction could not find any difference in the rates before and after the CCU was established.[41] Yet the researchers who reported these results concluded their report with the statement: "However, despite the relative paucity of impressive benefits, the CCU is a valuable addition to the therapy of myocardial infarction. In our hospital [the site of the study] it yielded dividends in medical care, education and research that warranted the investment in space, staffing, and the required electronic hardware."[42]

40. A. L. Cochrane, *Effectiveness and Efficiency: Random Reflections on Health Services* (London: Nuffield Provincial Hospitals Trust, 1972); A. Colling, "Home or Hospital Care after Myocardial Infarction: Is this the Right Question?" *British Medical Journal,* vol. 1 (March 23, 1974), pp. 559–63.

41. I. Donald Fagin and K. M. Anandiah, "The Coronary Care Unit and Mortality from Myocardial Infarction: A Continued Evaluation," *Journal of the American Geriatrics Society,* vol. 19 (August 1971), pp. 675–86.

42. Ibid., p. 685.

An even more striking example is given by A. L. Cochrane, who, in his discussion of the British study that compared home and hospital care, writes:

The first report after a few months of the trial showed a slightly greater death-rate in those treated in hospital than in those treated at home. Some one reversed the figures and showed them to a CCU enthusiast who immediately declared that the trial was unethical, and must be stopped at once. When, however, he was shown the table the correct way round he could not be persuaded to declare CCUs unethical![43]

In the emotionally charged atmosphere of medical care, the momentum of a new technology too often puts the burden of proof on those who question the evidence for it, rather than on those who propose it. The result is that the technology quickly becomes the accepted thing to do. Once it is, further attempts to test it are subject to the charge of being unethical, because a proper test requires that some patients not be given the by-now accepted treatment.

But even without the perfect test, it is clear that the benefits of intensive care are fairly small. It is not like penicillin, a therapy with results so consistent and impressive that no controlled trial was needed.[44] The benefits of intensive care are of a lower order of magnitude: a reduction in complications for certain groups of patients and, perhaps, reduced mortality for others.[45] Its costs are of the first order of magnitude.

This is the kind of specific problem that makes up the larger question: How much do we want to spend on medical care? The billions of dollars spent on intensive care each year probably bring some benefit to some people. Do we think these benefits merit the continued expenditure or the inevitable, under present circumstances, growth in that expenditure? If not, how much expenditure does it merit and for which patients? What we spend on medical care is the result of the decisions we make, or avoid making, about questions like these.

43. Cochrane, *Effectiveness and Efficiency*, p. 53.
44. Ibid., p. 30.
45. In some instances, this may be an equivocal benefit, because the life saved is so hampered by mental and physical handicaps; see, for example, the discussion of neonatal intensive care in A. R. Jonsen and others, "Critical Issues in Newborn Intensive Care: A Conference Report and Policy Proposal," *Pediatrics*, vol. 55 (June 1975), pp. 756–68.

chapter four **The Speed of Diffusion of**
Three Technologies

The technologies considered in this chapter—respiratory therapy, diagnostic radioisotopes, and the electroencephalograph—share two characteristics: a large number of metropolitan hospitals adopted them for the first time during the years from 1961 to 1975; and they were included in the American Hospital Association's surveys during enough of those years to capture much or all of the diffusion. The analysis in this chapter analyzes the AHA data to try to identify the factors that influenced the speed of diffusion of these technologies, with speed measured by the number of years it took different hospitals to adopt them.

Figures 4-1, 4-2, and 4-3 show the national trends for private non-profit community hospitals. Respiratory therapy departments, which collect under one organizational heading the technically dissimilar therapies aimed at the treatment of respiratory conditions, spread very fast during the 1960s. By the time the AHA first included them in the survey, in 1968, their diffusion was nearly complete among hospitals of 200 beds or more, and they were well established among smaller ones (figure 4-1).

The survey has followed the diagnostic use of radioisotopes and the electroencephalograph (a device for measuring the electrical activity of the brain) for a much longer period, beginning in the early 1950s.[1] Of the two, diagnostic radioisotopes were adopted more enthusiastically, and by 1960 there were not many large hospitals (300 beds or more) that did not have facilities for them. Although its diffusion was farther along in 1953 than that of diagnostic radioisotopes, the electroencephalograph was adopted more slowly in the following years, and a sizable number of large hospitals still had not adopted it by 1960. The adoption of both technologies by smaller hospitals picked up noticeably in the late 1960s.

1. Since the surveys for years before 1961 are not on tape, it was not possible to include those years in the statistical analysis.

Figure 4-1. Percent of Private Nonprofit Hospitals with Respiratory Therapy Departments, by Size of Hospital, 1968–76

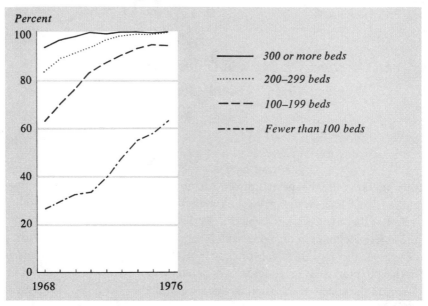

Sources: *Hospitals, Journal of the American Hospital Association,* vol. 45 (August 1, 1971), Guide Issue, pt. 2, and preceding annual guide issues; *Hospital Statistics,* annual issues.

The hospitals used in the statistical analysis were drawn from the same group that provided the base for analyzing the speed of diffusion of intensive care. These are the 2,770 hospitals that were in metropolitan areas —based on the 1975 definitions of metropolitan areas—and that answered the AHA survey in at least ten of the fifteen years between 1961 and 1975. The group produced 712 hospitals that adopted respiratory therapy, 880 that adopted diagnostic radioisotopes, and 1,006 that adopted electroencephalography during the period.

The distributions of these hospitals by year of adoption (table 4-1) are consistent with the national trends.[2] The number reporting respiratory therapy for the first time starts out high in 1969 and declines quickly for more recent years, as the process of diffusion neared completion; since most large hospitals had already established departments by the late 1960s, only about 20 percent of the adopters in the study group are

2. The distributions start in each case with the second year in which the technology appeared on the tapes. It was impossible to distinguish new adopters in the first year—1968 in the case of respiratory therapy, 1961 for diagnostic radioisotopes and the electroencephalograph—from hospitals that had adopted earlier.

hospitals with 200 beds or more (table 4-2). The diffusion of diagnostic radioisotopes is spread more evenly over the period, but here, too, few of the adopters are large hospitals. Both distributions, by year of adoption and by size, confirm the slower spread of the electroencephalograph.

Like the preceding and following chapters, this one presents brief sketches of each of the technologies—their histories, what they are used for, their costs and their benefits—before turning to the statistical analysis. While they are dissimilar in many respects, they are also alike in several ways besides their overlapping diffusion spans. For one thing, all three are quite common, so common that questions of geographic accessibility really do not arise, as they do for rarer technologies, such as those considered in chapter 5; so many hospitals have them that they are almost always available nearby. They are also low-risk, and this may account in part for their commonness: where the risks are high, there is more pressure for the technology to be limited to centers with the expertise to handle it well. Finally, their costs per procedure are relatively low; but their aggregate costs are substantial, both because so many hospitals have them, and because each hospital uses them so often.

Figure 4-2. Percent of Private Nonprofit Hospitals with Diagnostic Radioisotope Facilities, by Size of Hospital, 1953-76[a]

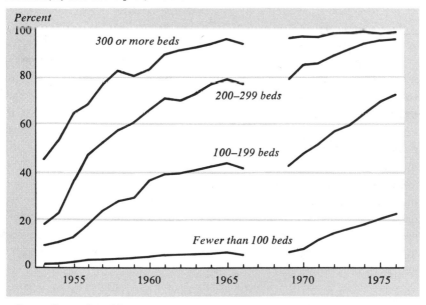

Sources: Same as figure 4-1.
a. Gaps in the lines reflect years in which the facility was omitted from the survey.

Figure 4-3. Percent of Private Nonprofit Hospitals with Electroencephalographs, by Size of Hospital, 1953–76[a]

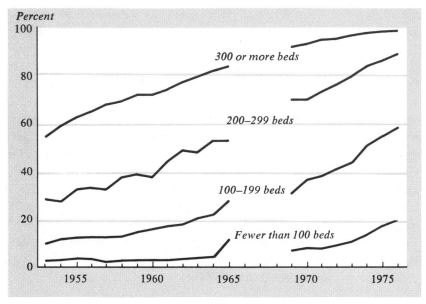

Sources: Same as figure 4-1.
a. Gaps in the lines reflect years in which the facility was omitted from the survey.

Respiratory Therapy

Respiratory therapy, and respiratory therapy departments, encompass a range of services used in the diagnosis and treatment of patients with respiratory conditions. There are four major types of therapy: the use of oxygen and oxygen mixtures; the use of humidity and aerosol mists to keep the respiratory tract moist and to administer medications; chest physical therapy, which includes exercises to reduce the effort of breathing and tapping and coughing procedures to help clear the lungs; and the use of mechanical ventilators to replace in whole or in part the spontaneous breathing of the patient. To diagnose problems, respiratory therapy departments make use of a variety of tests to determine the levels of oxygen and carbon dioxide in the blood, the volume of air taken into the lungs, and so on; often the department will have its own laboratory in which to carry out these tests.[3]

3. Stanton Belinkoff, *Introduction to Inhalation Therapy* (Little, Brown, 1969); Donald F. Egan, "Inhalation Therapy Department: Staffing and Services," *Hospitals, Journal of the American Hospital Association,* vol. 42 (September 1, 1968), pp. 40–47.

Table 4-1. Distributions of Study Hospitals by Year Technology Was Adopted, 1962-75[a]

| | Number and percent of hospitals adopting technology | | | | | |
| | Respiratory therapy | | Diagnostic radioisotopes | | Electroencephalograph | |
Year	Number	Percent	Number	Percent	Number	Percent
1962	...	...	41	4.7	41	4.1
1963	...	...	54	6.1	68	6.8
1964	...	...	52	5.9	76	7.6
1965	...	...	53	6.0	86	8.5
1966	...	...	51	5.8	...	...
1967	...	...	...	...	...	...
1968	...	...	...	...	...	...
1969	211	29.6	172	19.5	274	27.2
1970	116	16.3	84	9.5	84	8.3
1971	127	17.8	81	9.2	80	8.0
1972	81	11.4	84	9.5	70	7.0
1973	70	9.8	73	8.3	75	7.5
1974	56	7.9	58	6.6	71	7.1
1975	51	7.2	77	8.8	81	8.1
Total	712	100.0	880	100.0	1,006	100.0

Sources: American Hospital Association's surveys 1961-75; only metropolitan hospitals that responded to at least ten of the fifteen surveys were included in the study group. Figures are rounded.

a. The years for which no data are shown are years when the technology was omitted from the survey. Hospitals that adopted diagnostic radioisotopes in 1967-68 and electroencephalographs in 1966-68 are counted in 1969, their first chance to report.

Singly or in combination, these therapies are used for virtually every kind of respiratory problem seen in hospitals. They are often prescribed to treat, or with the intention of preventing, the respiratory complications that sometimes follow trauma, poisoning, or surgery, especially major surgery like open-heart procedures and organ transplants. People with the chronic lung diseases—principally asthma, bronchitis, and emphysema—

Table 4-2. Distributions of Study Hospitals Adopting Technology, by Size, 1962-75

| | Number and percent of hospitals adopting technology | | | | | |
| Beds in hospital[a] | Respiratory therapy | | Diagnostic radioisotopes | | Electroencephalograph | |
	Number	Percent	Number	Percent	Number	Percent
Under 100	326	45.8	215	24.4	191	19.0
100-199	240	33.7	389	44.2	333	33.1
200-299	82	11.5	200	22.7	286	28.4
300 and over	64	9.0	76	8.6	196	19.5
Total	712	100.0	880	100.0	1,006	100.0

Sources: Same as table 4-1.
a. Number of beds in year of adoption, or if not available, the year before or after.

undergo treatment to ease their discomfort and breathing problems.[4]
These diseases were the ninth-ranked cause of death in the United States
in the early 1970s.[5]

A fairly extensive review of the literature published in the last ten years
failed to turn up any evidence that a new invention or medical break-
through has been responsible for the boom in respiratory therapy. In fact,
many of the therapies—oxygen, mechanical ventilators, and aerosols, for
example—have been around for years. What is new is their organization
into a single department and their recent surge of growth.[6]

There is plenty of evidence to demonstrate the growth of respiratory
therapy. At the Yale-New Haven Hospital, for example, the proportion of
patients admitted to the hospital who received some form of respiratory
therapy during their stay rose from 10 percent in 1961–62 to 19 percent
in 1966–67.[7] Several more recent reports indicate that in some hospitals
25 or 30 percent of all admissions are given respiratory therapy.[8] The
number of people treated as outpatients can add substantially to the total:
one 680-bed hospital reported as early as 1970 that its department averaged twenty outpatient visits a day and also provided services for patients
in nursing homes and at home.[9]

Although charges for respiratory therapy can be substantial for those

4. Grant Fletcher, "Should Your Hospital Have an Inhalation Therapy Service?" *Hospital Practice,* vol. 3 (May 1968), pp. 47–53; William J. Monagle and
Evelyn L. Cassara, "Report Tells How 'Fastest Growing' Hospital Specialty Got
That Way," *Modern Hospital,* vol. 115 (November 1970), pp. 74–77; Thomas L.
Petty and others, "Intensive Respiratory Care Unit: Review of Ten Years' Experience," *Journal of the American Medical Association,* vol. 233 (July 7, 1975), pp.
34–37.

5. Gerald N. Olsen and others, "A Survey of Respiratory Care Resources in
Florida," *Journal of the Florida Medical Association,* vol. 61 (June 1974), pp.
437–44.

6. Frederick W. Cheney, Jr., "Is Your Respiratory Care Unit Up to Snuff?"
Resident and Staff Physician, vol. 22 (January 1976), pp. 66–69; Jean Maunsell,
"How One 250-bed Hospital Set Up an I.T. Department," *Hospital Administration
in Canada,* vol. 12 (September 1970), pp. 33–34; Monagle and Cassara, "Report
Tells How 'Fastest Growing' Hospital Specialty Got That Way."

7. Egan, "Inhalation Therapy Department."

8. George G. Burton and others, "Respiratory Care Warrants Studies for Cost-
Effectiveness," *Hospitals, Journal of the American Hospital Association,* vol. 49
(November 16, 1975), pp. 61 ff.; Fletcher, "Should Your Hospital Have an Inhala-
tion Therapy Service?"; Philip Leeber, Charles Cook, and William L. Sawyer,
"Contracting Respiratory Therapy Care," *Hospital Topics,* vol. 53 (January–Feb-
ruary 1975), pp. 6–7.

9. Monagle and Cassara, "Report Tells How 'Fastest Growing' Hospital Specialty Got That Way."

who receive it, especially if they are inpatients,[10] the expense involved appears to be more often a matter of a large number of procedures than high cost per procedure. For example, an intermittent positive pressure breathing (IPPB) procedure, in which a mechanical ventilator is used to assist the patient's breathing for twenty to thirty minutes, was generally priced below $15 in 1975.[11] But these procedures are typically prescribed at a rate of three or four times a day per patient, over several days or weeks.[12] They form the largest single item in most respiratory departments' workloads and are done in enormous quantities. A 1973 survey of 118 hospitals found that the number of IPPBs averaged 1,000 per month in hospitals with 100 through 199 beds (12,000 a year) and increased with size to 6,000 per month in hospitals with 500 beds or more (72,000 a year).[13]

The American Hospital Association estimates that, as of 1972, respiratory therapy services accounted for about 1 percent of total hospital costs,[14] certainly nothing on the scale of intensive care costs (see chapter 3) but nonetheless significant and, more important, growing fast: the 1972 percentage was almost 50 percent greater than the percentage for 1969. In dollar terms, the costs in fiscal 1972 were approximately $330 million, with community hospitals accounting for about $260 million of the total. There are no percentage estimates for more recent years, but had the percentage been the same in 1975 as in 1972, the costs of respiratory therapy would have been $470 million, with $390 million of the amount spent by community hospitals. Had costs of respiratory therapy increased another 50 percent over those three years, to 1.5 percent of hospital costs, they would have totaled $700 million, $590 million being spent by community hospitals.[15]

10. Burton and others, "Respiratory Care Warrants Studies for Cost-Effectiveness."

11. Dodie Gust, "Looming on the Horizon: Time and Cost Accounting in RT," *Respiratory Therapy,* vol. 5 (July–August 1975), pp. 45–48.

12. Donald F. Egan, *Fundamentals of Respiratory Therapy,* 2nd ed. (Mosby, 1973), p. 433.

13. James P. Baker, "Magnitude of Usage of Intermittent Positive Pressure Breathing," in *Proceedings of the Conference on the Scientific Basis of Respiratory Therapy,* pt. 2 of *American Review of Respiratory Disease,* vol. 110 (December 1974), pp. 170–77.

14. "Administrative Profiles: Anesthesiology, Inhalation Therapy, and Physical Therapy," *Hospitals, Journal of the American Hospital Association,* vol. 47 (May 16, 1973), p. 30.

15. Costs for all hospitals were derived by applying the percentages to the national costs of hospital care in Marjorie Smith Mueller and Robert M. Gibson,

The Joint Commission on the Accreditation of Hospitals (JCAH), the long-established guardian of standards in the hospital field, set its first standards for respiratory therapy services in January 1974. The discussion surrounding the introduction of the standards brought out a number of criticisms of respiratory therapy: that many physicians knew little about it and effectively turned therapeutic decisions over to the department staff; that techniques varied from hospital to hospital, and even within hospitals; and that some departments pushed quantity to the detriment of quality (one panel agreed that, although twenty to twenty-five IPPBs were as many as a therapist could do well in an eight-hour day, they knew of departments where the average was forty or more).[16] The JCAH standards tried to address some of these problems by, for example, requiring that the physician's order for services indicate the criteria for continuing or ending the therapeutic procedures to be used.[17]

But the criticism of respiratory therapy goes farther than this, to raise serious questions about its value for the patient even in the best of departments. A conference held in May 1974 considered the use of respiratory therapy for patients with chronic lung disease. The conference editors observed that the field had developed empirically, on the basis of hunch and clinical impression, and that there had not been enough testing. Reviewing the evidence that had accumulated, the contributors produced these critical findings:

Use of bland aerosols, particularly mist tents, in the treatment of lower respiratory disease was reviewed and no convincing evidence of efficacy was found. . . . Mist tents may be detrimental, in some cases, because of bacterial contamination and because they can cause bronchospasm.[18]

For patients with COPD [chronic obstructive pulmonary disease] stabilized in a treatment program that includes bronchodilator, adequate H_2O intake,

---

"National Health Expenditures, Fiscal Year 1975," *Social Security Bulletin,* vol. 39 (February 1976), p. 12; costs for community hospitals were derived by applying the same percentages to the costs for these hospitals in American Hospital Association, *Hospital Statistics, 1976 Edition: Data from the American Hospital Association 1975 Annual Survey.* Since respiratory therapy is given to many intensive care patients, the costs of intensive care (discussed in chapter 3) include some respiratory therapy costs and the two cost estimates are not mutually exclusive.

16. Bob Skalnik, "IPPB: A Question of Quality," *Respiratory Therapy,* vol. 6 (November–December 1976), pp. 81–83, 110.

17. Cheney, "Is Your Respiratory Care Unit Up to Snuff?"

18. Lewis E. Gibson, "Use of Water Vapor in the Treatment of Lower Respiratory Disease," *Proceedings of the Conference on the Scientific Basis of Respiratory Therapy,* p. 100.

bronchial toilet, and antibiotic drugs when necessary, . . . adding routine administration of aerosolized mucolytic agent . . . is of neither subjective nor objective benefit.[19]

. . . owing to the lack of evidence to support the widespread application of IPPB and the costs and possible hazards of this modality of treatment, it is recommended that further use of IPPB in patients with stable COPD be discouraged. . . .[20]

It is hard to prove that a procedure does absolutely no one any good. It is always possible that if the sample were larger a statistically significant benefit would appear;[21] or that a small number of patients are benefiting a great deal, but the effect is lost because they are averaged with a large group who are not. One of the natural reactions to the criticisms, then, is that what is needed is further trials with more carefully standardized therapeutic techniques. Others accept some of the conclusions but see the shape rather than the size of respiratory therapy changing (one hospital has replaced the routine use of IPPBs after surgery with a program of aerosol therapy, deep-breathing exercises, and frequent turning and changing of position). Another authority believes that IPPBs have benefits but that these can be achieved by the alternate route of teaching the patient breathing exercises, cough control, and other special techniques.[22]

As in the case of intensive care, it seems safe to say that the benefits of this technology, or group of technologies, are fairly small, their costs— at least in the aggregate—fairly large. Better tests of its efficacy can make this conclusion more precise by identifying more precisely who it is that benefits and how. But even with better studies, the more difficult question remains. The philosophy expressed by third party payment is that no benefit is too small or too costly. Given the expenditures required to support this philosophy, and the evidence that the returns from those expenditures can indeed be quite small and quite costly, do we want to continue to support it? If not, where are we willing to draw the line?

19. A. Don Barton, "Aerosolized Detergents and Mucolytic Agents in the Treatment of Stable Chronic Obstructive Pulmonary Disease," ibid., p. 104.

20. John F. Murray, "Review of the State of the Art in Intermittent Positive Pressure Breathing Therapy," ibid., p. 193.

21. A. L. Cochrane observes that a large enough sample can produce a result that is statistically significant but "clinically unimportant," that is, not large enough to matter (*Effectiveness and Efficiency: Random Reflections on Health Services* [London: Nuffield Provincial Hospitals Trust, 1972], p. 23).

22. Skalnik, "IPPB: A Question of Quality."

Diagnostic Radioisotopes

Nuclear medicine is the branch of radiology that uses radioisotopes—unstable atoms that give off radiation spontaneously—in diagnosis and therapy. The diagnostic applications are far more voluminous and widespread, and this aspect of nuclear medicine has been included in the AHA survey for many years. (The therapeutic uses of radioisotopes in implants and injections, first added to the survey in 1971, are not discussed in this section.)

The medical usefulness of radioisotopes arises from the correspondence between their physiological properties and those of the stable version of the same elements: they combine with the same substances and concentrate in the same organs. When a radioisotope is injected into the patient or is taken by mouth, its radioactivity can be detected from outside and monitored to describe various characteristics and functions of the parts of the body in which it settles. For example, in the normal brain the blood–brain barrier keeps radioactive substances in the blood from being absorbed by the tissue, but in areas of disease this barrier breaks down and diseased areas show up on the scan as concentrations of radioactivity.[23]

A scan can be produced by a rectilinear scanner or by a scintillation camera, sometimes referred to as a nuclear camera. The rectilinear scanner moves across the patient's body in a series of parallel lines, and the early models produced a map—by means of a mechanical printer—of the amount of radiation detected at each location in the body. Most modern scanners produce a film, but often use the printed record as well, as a way of allowing the operator to follow the progress of the scan. Invented more recently (in 1958) the scintillation camera works on the same principle as the scanner—both are activated by the light flashes produced as the radiation strikes a sodium iodide crystal—but the camera produces a film of the pattern of radiation without having to scan the patient physically. A device called a well-counter is used for test-tube studies: a test tube of

23. Arif Azam, "Radionuclide Organ Imaging (Scanning)," *Medical Trial Technique Quarterly,* vol. 22 (Summer 1975), pp. 78–88; D. N. Croft and Olwen Williams, "Radioisotopes in Clinical Practice," *British Journal of Clinical Practice,* vol. 23 (December 1969), pp. 493–500.

the substance to be examined, such as blood, is taken from the patient and put in the counter to measure its radioactivity.[24]

The ability of these instruments to detect and record the course of the radioisotope in the patient is important, but the choice of a radioisotope is critical, and progress in the field has been very much a matter of finding, or more often, producing, radioisotopes with appropriate combinations of characteristics. (Most radioisotopes used in medicine do not occur in nature but are created in linear accelerators by bombarding the stable isotope of the element with high-energy particles or radiation.) To be useful, a radioisotope must have an affinity for the organ of the body to be studied and, usually, a tendency to be taken up more readily by either the healthy or the diseased parts of the organ so that the two can be differentiated. Or it must be taken up by a substance that follows a circulatory, metabolic, or excretory pathway through the body; for example, blood tagged with a radioisotope can trace through the circulatory system, revealing blocked vessels as it goes. The radioactive life of the isotope, which is denoted by its half-life and can vary from a few seconds to hundreds of years, must be long enough to allow it to reach the organ and send out signals but not so long as to present a danger from radiation if it remains inside the patient. Isotopes with long half-lives can nevertheless be used if they are eliminated fairly quickly from the body. Finally, isotopes that produce gamma radiation are preferred because they penetrate the body better and are easier to track than isotopes that produce beta radiation, even though this means they are also more dangerous.[25]

Isotopes capable of producing useful information about thyroid function were among the first to be discovered. By the mid-1960s, isotopes had been identified that permitted scans of the brain, thyroid, lungs, heart, liver, spleen, pancreas, kidneys, and bones. These tests are generally used in the diagnosis of tumors and other space-occupying processes, such as embolisms and abscesses. For cancer they can be useful not only in the initial diagnosis but in testing whether the tumor has spread, in locating

24. Hal O. Anger, "The Instruments of Nuclear Medicine: I," *Hospital Practice,* vol. 7 (June 1972), pp. 45–54; Azam, "Radionuclide Organ Imaging"; Edward M. Dwyer, Jr., "Radioisotope Studies in Coronary Artery Disease," *Cardiovascular Clinics,* vol. 7, no. 2 (1975), pp. 101–12; Robert N. Beck, "The Instruments of Nuclear Medicine: II," *Hospital Practice,* vol. 7 (July 1972), pp. 57–68; D. W. Hill, "Progress in Medical Instrumentation over the Past Fifty Years," *Journal of Scientific Instruments,* vol. 1 (July 1968), pp. 697–701.

25. Azam, "Radionuclide Organ Imaging"; Dwyer, "Radioisotope Studies."

the tumor precisely (important for the planning of radiotherapy), and in checking the success of treatment. Other nuclear medicine procedures can be used to measure blood or red blood-cell volume, to test red blood-cell survival, and to test iron metabolism. Dynamic function studies include tests to measure the intestine's ability to absorb or tendency to lose substances, and tests to measure kidney function and drainage.[26]

The advantages of radioisotope procedures are that they are low-risk and noninvasive: the patient does not have to be cut open. Radiation risk is small; Azam states that, over the three decades of nuclear medicine's development, there have been no reports of tissue damage or genetic mutation caused by the procedures. The disadvantage is that the tests are not specific to particular diseases; that is, they show that something is wrong and outline its location, but they are less helpful in identifying the disease or condition responsible for the problem.[27]

The advantages of the diagnostic uses of radioisotopes have been enough to stimulate rapid growth. Between 1971 and 1975, the number of nuclear medicine procedures per 100 hospital admissions almost doubled, from 11.7 to 22.2.[28] Brain scans were a major portion of the total. These tests provide as much information as the X-ray techniques more often used in the 1960s, which involved injecting materials opaque to radiation into the brain cavity, and are considerably safer.[29] A 1973 survey of six hospitals in California found that brain scans accounted for more than a third of the procedures performed, while together with liver scans, thyroid

26. Azam, "Radionuclide Organ Imaging"; Merrill A. Bender, "Should your Hospital Have a Nuclear Medicine Unit?" *Hospital Practice,* vol. 2 (February 1967), pp. 43–53; Croft and Williams, "Radioisotopes in Clinical Practice"; George G. Green, "Present State of Isotope Procedures," *West Virginia Medical Journal,* vol. 61 (July 1965), pp. 163–65; William D. Kaplan and S. James Adelstein, "The Radionuclide Identification of Tumors," *Cancer,* vol. 37 (January 1976), supplement, pp. 487–95.

27. Azam, "Radionuclide Organ Imaging"; N. T. Bateman and D. N. Croft, "False-Positive Lung Scans and Radiotherapy," *British Medical Journal,* vol. 1 (April 3, 1976), pp. 807–08; Edward B. Silberstein, "Cancer Diagnosis: The Role of Tumor-Imaging Radiopharmaceuticals," *American Journal of Medicine,* vol. 60 (February 1976), pp. 226–37.

28. William A. Michela, "Administrative Profiles: Trends in the Volumes of Services Utilized," *Hospitals, Journal of the American Hospital Association,* vol. 50 (September 1, 1976), p. 55. Although the article does not say so, the data probably include the relatively small number of therapeutic procedures as well as diagnostic ones.

29. Bender, "Should your Hospital Have a Nuclear Medicine Unit?"; Croft and Williams, "Radioisotopes in Clinical Practice"; Green, "Present State of Isotope Procedures."

scans, and thyroid uptakes (a test of thyroid function), they made up 72 percent of the survey hospitals' volume.[30]

Nothing stands still in medical technology. In the middle 1970s diagnostic nuclear medicine suffered a setback because of the introduction of the CT scanner. The early scanners were designed primarily for head studies and cut sharply into the use of radioisotope brain scans. But the setback was brief. Among other developments, new methods for dynamic studies of heart function—in which a lump of radioactive material is recorded as it travels through the heart and large blood vessels—have helped keep diagnostic nuclear medicine growing as fast as ever. These dynamic studies can often be used in place of the far more dangerous procedure of cardiac catheterization to study the condition of the heart before open-heart surgery and to evaluate the success of the operation afterwards.[31]

In terms of the initial investment and the cost per procedure, diagnostic radioisotope procedures are not particularly expensive. In 1973, a scintillation camera cost about $55,000. A rectilinear scanner and a wellcounter—which are sufficient for the performance of the simpler studies—together cost less than $20,000.[32] The equipment necessary to update a scintillation camera for dynamic heart function studies cost, in 1977, between $25,000 and $40,000.[33] The most expensive procedure in 1973, based on the California relative value scale, was the brain scan at $120;[34] the cost of the drug is often the largest part of the expense for a radioisotope test.[35] The new dynamic heart-function studies were estimated at about $150 each in 1977, much less than the cost of a cardiac catheterization.[36]

30. N. Jeanne Harris and Leslie R. Bennett, "Planning a Nuclear Medicine Service," *Hospitals, Journal of the American Hospital Association,* vol. 47 (October 1, 1973), pp. 90–94, and ibid. (October 16, 1973), pp. 84–94. The remaining 28 percent of the total consisted of lung scans (8 percent), bone scans (5 percent), kidney scans (5 percent), and a miscellaneous group of other procedures (10 percent).

31. Dwyer, "Radioisotope Studies"; Liz Roman Gallese, "Viewing the Heart: Nuclear Scans Improve Diagnosis, Treatment of Cardiovascular Ills," *Wall Street Journal,* November 9, 1977.

32. Harris and Bennett, "Planning a Nuclear Medicine Service."

33. Gallese, "Viewing the Heart."

34. Harris and Bennett, "Planning a Nuclear Medicine Service."

35. John W. Hamilton, "A Method for Estimating the Cost, Growth Rate and Efficiency of Radioisotope Laboratories," *American Journal of Medical Technology,* vol. 34 (August 1968), pp. 473–81.

36. Gallese, "Viewing the Heart."

The contribution of diagnostic radioisotopes to hospital costs is nevertheless important because of its high volume and capacity for further growth. A very rough estimate puts the cost of the procedures performed in community hospitals at about $630 million in 1975, or 1.6 percent of their total costs.[37] If the same percentage applied to all hospitals—a reasonable assumption for federal short-term hospitals but less reasonable for the long-term and psychiatric hospitals that complete the total— the costs were closer to $780 million.

The reports about the new heart studies suggest the scope for future growth. Not only will many of these tests be done to check on suspected problems or on the outcome of surgery in cases where catheterization would not have been done, because of the risk, but there is speculation that these tests, or variants of them, may become standard screening devices, perhaps even a routine part of the physical examination.

The Electroencephalograph

The electroencephalograph (EEG) is a machine used in diagnosis and monitoring that measures the electrical activity of the brain. The standard technique for using it is noninvasive: the electrodes that are part of the machine are placed on the patient's scalp to pick up the electrical activity that reaches the surface, and this is recorded for thirty minutes to an hour, resulting in 180 to 360 pages of continuous graphs (the electroencephalo- *gram*) of the voltage measured at each electrode location. To try to tease out abnormalities, the patient is recorded under varying conditions: asleep

37. The estimate is derived by multiplying the level of procedures in 1975 (22.2 per 100 admissions) by the number of admissions to nonfederal short-term hospitals in 1975 (33,519,000) and an average charge of $85 for 1973 based on the California relative value scale. The level of procedures may be slightly overstated by the inclusion of therapeutic radioisotope procedures. The use of the California charge is based on the assumptions that, while California was undoubtedly more costly than the average in 1973, the average had caught up to that number by 1975, and that the national distribution of procedures by type was similar to that in California; the number is from Harris and Bennett, "Planning a Nuclear Medicine Service." Admissions and total costs for community hospitals and all hospitals are from *Hospital Statistics, 1976 Edition: Data from the American Hospital Association 1975 Annual Survey*. As a final caveat, it should be noted that charges are not the same as costs; in the case of an ancillary service like nuclear medicine, charges are likely to be higher. Thus the average 1973 California charge almost certainly overstates the 1973 cost, although it may not overstate 1975 costs.

(or sedated), awake, while hyperventilated, while being subjected to flashing light and, sometimes, after convulsant drugs have been administered. The recording is then summarized in terms of the duration, amplitude, and form of the wave patterns that appear and of the points on the scalp that produced those patterns.[38]

Like diagnostic radioisotope procedures (and most other diagnostic procedures, for that matter), the results of an EEG are generally not specific to a particular disease. Most conditions show up the same way—as an unusual amount of the slower rhythms and a depression of normal rhythms in a particular area of the brain, reflecting a reduction in the oxygen supply to that area. Although the hope has always been that it is possible to associate distinct wave forms with particular diseases, this approach has not met with much success. Even the rhythms that commonly appear in recordings of the normal brain do not provide the kind of consistent baseline—both for different people, and for the same person at different times—that the rhythms of the heart do for electrocardiograph recordings, for example, and the deviations from these normal rhythms can seldom be linked to a specific disease. The outstanding exception is seizure disorders, especially epilepsy, which often produce a characteristic spike pattern. But as a general rule, the primary value of the EEG in diagnosis is that it can determine that *some* problem exists, and, if the problem is localized, help to describe its position in the brain.[39]

The use of the EEG is not much discussed in the medical literature and, when it is, the statements suggest that the test has some value but that it is hemmed in by substitute tests and by its own limitations. The crosscurrents are indicated by one authority's assessment that the use of the EEG is declining in some areas—the location of cerebral lesions and space-occupying processes in particular—but increasing in others, such

38. Richard N. Harner, "Principles of EEG Evaluation, Interpretation, and Reporting," *American Journal of EEG Technology,* vol. 14 (December 1974), pp. 211–17; James A. Lewis, "Electroencephalography: The Lab Test That Nobody Knows," *Resident and Staff Physician,* vol. 20 (June 1974), pp. 47–56; Donald H. Pellar, "Recent Advances in Neurodiagnostic Laboratory Procedures: I. Electroencephalography, Electromyography and Echoencephalography," *Modern Treatment,* vol. 8 (May 1971), pp. 288–301.

39. Harner, "Principles of EEG Evaluation"; Lewis, "Electroencephalography"; P. J. O'Connor, "The Value of Routine Electroencephalography," *Practitioner,* vol. 211 (August 1973), pp. 178–81; Pellar, "Recent Advances in Neurodiagnostic Laboratory Procedures"; Harold W. Shipton, "EEG Analysis: A History and a Prospectus," *Annual Review of Biophysics and Bioengineering,* vol. 4 (1975), pp. 1–13.

as the detection of brain disease associated with liver malfunction.[40] One physician states, "Most of us have discarded the electroencephalogram in routine clinical use,"[41] while another argues that the EEG is still very useful in the diagnosis of such conditions as tumors and abscesses involving the hemispheric surface of the brain.[42]

Yet the electroencephalograph has continued to spread quite rapidly among hospitals of fewer than 300 beds, many of which have adopted it only in the last ten years (figure 4-3). The reason almost certainly lies in its more general usefulness as a monitoring device, in particular its use as the accepted way to establish brain death. Now that there are machines that can maintain the patient's circulation and respiration when he can no longer do so himself, some other method is necessary to determine that the patient is, if not dead in the strictest sense of the word, at least beyond hope of recovery. That method is the EEG. It is generally agreed that if the EEG is flat (isoelectric) for twelve to twenty-four hours—that is, if it shows no sign of rhythmic activity—then brain death has occurred. This has two important implications for treatment: it means that intensive care can be ended; and if the patient has agreed that one or more of his organs can be taken for transplant after his death, the organs can be removed.[43]

The growth of intensive care will undoubtedly help to stimulate the further growth of electroencephalography. But its status as one of the less known among the spreading technologies is clear from the title of one article, "Electroencephalography: The Lab Test That Nobody Knows,"[44] and is reflected in the fact that, while it is included in the AHA survey, and has been for many years, there are almost no data on the volume of procedures, the growth in that volume, the relative importance of different uses, or the costs associated with them.

What little information there is indicates that the investment costs and costs per procedure of electroencephalography are not great. A British unit reported that the machine itself could be purchased for about $7,500

40. E. Niedermeyer, "Progress and Crisis—The Present State of Clinical Electroencephalography," *American Journal of EEG Technology,* vol. 15 (March 1975), pp. 1–13.

41. "Computers in Anesthesiology and Intensive Care," *Acta Anaesthesiologica Belgica,* vol. 23 (1975), supplement, p. 245.

42. Lewis, "Electroencephalography."

43. Ibid.; Daniel Silverman and others, "Cerebral Death and the Electroencephalogram: Report of the Ad Hoc Committee of the American Electroencephalographic Society on EEG Criteria for Determination of Cerebral Death," *Journal of the American Medical Association,* vol. 209 (September 8, 1969), pp. 1505–10.

44. Lewis.

(£3,000) in 1973 but gave no idea of the possible range of machines and prices.[45] Major additional items of equipment may include one or more machines designed to help analyze the reams of paper produced by the EEG, and these can require a special-use computer or access to a general-use computer;[46] there is no indication of the proportion of units that have such machines. Record storage is an obvious problem and is sometimes, but apparently not often, based on tape systems.[47] The physical requirements for the EEG lab are modest, complicated only by the need to shield the lab against outside sources of electromagnetic interference; but many EEGs are done outside the lab—the machine is designed to be portable—where special space is not provided and special shielding not possible.[48]

Altogether, the electroencephalograph appears to be a technology that has been fairly stable on the technical side and has never quite fulfilled the early hopes for it. While its use is growing, it has managed to do so without attracting much attention, and the resulting dearth of information makes it impossible to attempt even a rough estimate of the total cost of electroencephalography.

The Statistical Analysis

The analysis discussed in this section tries to explain the speed of diffusion of each of the three technologies, or, put another way, the length of time it took different types of hospitals to adopt them. Of necessity, it focuses on the later adopters—hospitals that introduced respiratory therapy between 1968 and 1975 or diagnostic radioisotopes or the EEG between 1961 and 1975. These totaled 712 hospitals in 189 SMSAs for respiratory therapy, 880 hospitals in 201 SMSAs for diagnostic radioisotopes, and 1,006 hospitals in 225 SMSAs for the EEG. The analysis thus

45. O'Connor, "The Value of Routine Electroencephalography."

46. Shipton, "EEG Analysis."

47. J. S. Barlow and others, "EEG Instrumentation Standards: Report of the Committee on EEG Instrumentation Standards of the International Federation of Societies for Electroencephalography and Clinical Neurophysiology," *Electroencephalography and Clinical Neurophysiology,* vol. 37 (November 1974), pp. 549–53.

48. B. Echols Bucci, "Factors Affecting the Efficiency of EEG Laboratories of Varying Sizes," *American Journal of EEG Technology,* vol. 5 (June 1965), pp. 26–29; Nina Kagawa, "Laboratory Organization and Operation," ibid., vol. 1 (September 1961), pp. 75–84; Mary Lou Montoya and Gladys Hill, "EEG Recording in Intensive Care Units," ibid., vol. 8 (September 1968), pp. 85–95.

covers an important segment of the diffusion process, but not all of it, and it is not always clear how the results would have been altered had it been possible to include adopters from the years before 1961.

It is evident from the regressions in tables 4-3, 4-4, and 4-5 that this limitation is important for respiratory therapy; only a few of the most obvious factors show any effect. While this outcome may reflect the larger reality, it seems more likely to be due to the sharply truncated sample. The span of years for which adoption could be determined is much shorter for respiratory therapy, extending only from 1968 to 1975. Further, the adopting hospitals are bunched in the early years of the period (table 4-1) and are concentrated as well in the smallest size group (table 4-2). There is thus relatively little variation among the hospitals in the number of years before adoption, and what there is is strongly related to scale.

For diagnostic radioisotopes and the EEG, both of which have more observations spread more evenly over more years, a larger and more varied group of explanatory factors is important. The lack of better evidence for respiratory therapy is unfortunate since, as the case study and the national trends in figure 4-1 indicate, it accounts for a growing share of hospital costs. But accepting that lack, the discussion gives little weight to most of the respiratory therapy results and emphasizes those for diagnostic radioisotopes and the EEG instead.

Two regressions—one with and one without third party payment—are shown for each technology in the tables. Their form and interpretation are the same as in the analysis of the diffusion of intensive care units (chapter 3). The explanatory factors and the classes into which they are divided are generally the same, the most noteworthy exception being that, because there were relatively few hospitals with large residency programs in the samples, residency training has been reduced to only two classes. As before, the year at the top of each column is the estimated year of adoption for hospitals with all the reference class characteristics. The rest of the estimates in each table give the differences in the length of time until adoption, measured in years and fractions of years, associated with characteristics other than those of the reference classes. For example, using the estimates in the first column of table 4-3, hospitals with all the reference characteristics introduced respiratory therapy in late 1971 (1971.65), on average, while hospitals of 300 beds or more, but with the reference characteristics in all other respects, adopted it early in 1970 $(1971.65 - 1.27 = 1970.38)$.

Table 4-3. The Year in Which Respiratory Therapy Was Adopted by a Hospital, 1968–75: Differences Associated with Selected Characteristics of the Hospital and Its Market[a]

Characteristic	Year	
	Regression excluding third party payment	*Regression including third party payment*
Year for hospitals with all the reference characteristics[b]	1971.65 (97.0)**	1971.49 (73.4)**
	Differences associated with size, control, and service	
Beds[c]		
Under 100	Reference class	Reference class
100–199	−0.57 (3.4)**	−0.56 (3.3)**
200–299	−0.85 (3.4)**	−0.86 (3.4)**
300 and over	−1.27 (4.1)**	−1.33 (4.1)**
Control		
Private nonprofit	Reference class	Reference class
State and local government	+0.71 (3.9)**	+0.78 (4.2)**
Private, profit	−0.24 (1.1)	−0.17 (0.8)
Service		
General	Reference class	Reference class
Specialized	+0.66 (2.0)**	+0.75 (2.3)**
	Differences associated with teaching and research	
Medical school affiliation		
Yes	+0.06 (0.2)	+0.09 (0.2)
No	Reference class	Reference class
Residency training program[c]		
Yes	−0.34 (1.6)	−0.36 (1.6)*
No	Reference class	Reference class
Research grants to hospitals, dollars per bed		
0	Reference class	Reference class
1–99	−0.39 (1.6)	−0.37 (1.4)
100–999	−0.07 (0.3)	+0.03 (0.1)
1,000 and over	−0.03 (0.1)	+0.20 (0.6)
	Differences associated with patient care	
Doctors per 1,000 beds		
Under 175	−0.06 (0.3)	−0.16 (0.6)
175–249	Reference class	Reference class
250 and over	+0.02 (0.1)	−0.03 (0.2)
Deaths from respiratory disease per 1,000 beds		
Under 20	−0.20 (1.1)	−0.10 (0.5)
20–29	Reference class	Reference class
30–39	−0.29 (1.5)	−0.20 (0.9)
40 and over	−0.16 (0.6)	−0.17 (0.6)

Table 4-3 (*continued*)

	Year	
Characteristic	*Regression excluding third party payment*	*Regression including third party payment*
Differences associated with market structure		
Percent of beds in four largest hospitals		
Under 50	Reference class	Reference class
50–79	+0.37 (1.6)	+0.45 (1.8)*
80–100	+0.22 (0.8)	+0.26 (0.9)
Market with fewer than four hospitals	−0.45 (1.2)	−0.30 (0.7)
Percent growth in population, 1960–70		
Under 15	Reference class	Reference class
15–24	+0.12 (0.6)	+0.19 (0.9)
25 and over	+0.01 (0.1)	−0.03 (0.1)
Percent of hospitals with respiratory therapy in 1968		
Under 45	−0.16 (0.7)	−0.07 (0.3)
45–59	−0.15 (0.7)	−0.08 (0.3)
60–74	Reference class	Reference class
75 and over	−0.02 (0.1)	+0.05 (0.2)
Differences associated with third party payment		
Percent of population with hospital insurance, 1963		
Under 65	...	+0.45 (1.0)
65–74	...	−0.08 (0.2)
75–84	...	+0.13 (0.4)
85 or over	...	Reference class
Percent growth in hospital insurance, 1961–71		
Under 10	...	+0.29 (0.7)
10–19	...	Reference class
20–29	...	−0.03 (0.1)
30 and over	...	−0.10 (0.3)
Percent of costs paid by Medicare		
Under 15	...	+0.16 (0.5)
15–19	...	−0.46 (1.9)*
20–24	...	Reference class
25–29	...	+0.30 (1.2)
30 and over	...	−0.07 (0.2)
Differences associated with regulation		
Effective year, certificate-of-need law		
1965–69	+0.03 (0.1)	−0.29 (0.7)
1970–73	−0.17 (1.0)	−0.34 (1.4)
1974–75 or no law	Reference class	Reference class
Regional medical program dollars per hospital		
Under 100,000	...	Reference class
100,000 and over	...	+0.09 (0.4)

Table 4-3 (*continued*)

| | Year | |
Characteristic	Regression excluding third party payment	Regression including third party payment
	Differences associated with regulation (continued)	
Area comprehensive health planning dollars per hospital		
0	...	−0.13 (0.5)
1–4,999	...	+0.37 (1.4)
5,000–14,999	...	Reference class
15,000 and over	...	−0.08 (0.4)
Summary statistic		
Number of observations	712	712
R^2	0.113	0.134
Corrected R^2	0.081	0.084
F and degrees of freedom [numerator, denominator]	3.36 [26, 685]	2.60 [40, 671]

Sources: See chapter 2 for discussion of the basic data.

* The difference is statistically significant at the 90 percent level of confidence or better, but less than the 95 percent level.

** The difference is statistically significant at the 95 percent level of confidence or better.

a. The numbers in parentheses are *t*-statistics.

b. This is the constant term of the regression and shows the estimated year of adoption for hospitals having all the reference characteristics. (See text for explanation of the notion of a reference class.) The values of the dependent variable used in the regressions ranged from 29 (for 1969) to 35 (for 1975), but the constant is expressed here in terms of the corresponding calendar year to make its interpretation more obvious. The *t*-statistic in this case applies not to the number shown but to the difference between that number and 1940 (to 1971.65 − 1940 = 31.65 in column 1, for example.)

c. In the year respiratory therapy was adopted, or, if not available, the year before or after.

Scale is uniformly important.[49] In every case large hospitals adopted the technology sooner than did small hospitals, and the larger the hospital the greater the difference.[50] The differences are smallest in the case of respiratory therapy (which, as just noted, produced a rather skewed sample; only a few large hospitals had not yet adopted respiratory therapy by 1968): hospitals of 300 beds or more introduced the technology about 1.3 years earlier than those with fewer than 100 beds. For electroencephalography, the difference between the two extreme size groups is about two years. For diagnostic radioisotopes, it is larger—about three

49. Here, as throughout the study, only regression coefficients that are statistically significant at the 90 percent level of confidence or better are described as "significant," "important," or, indeed, as differences. Reference is seldom made in the text to *t*-statistics or levels of significance, however, in order to keep the discussion as clear and readable as possible.

50. The most numerous class of any set was generally chosen to be the reference class, in order to reduce the collinearity among the variables in the regression. Since relatively fewer of the smallest hospitals adopted diagnostic radioisotopes or the EEG during the sample period (see table 4-2), hospitals with 100 through 199 beds were made the reference group in tables 4-4 and 4-5.

Table 4-4. The Year in Which Diagnostic Radioisotopes Were Adopted by a Hospital, 1961–75: Differences Associated with Selected Characteristics of the Hospital and Its Market[a]

Characteristic	Year	
	Regression excluding third party payment	Regression including third party payment
Year for hospitals with all the reference characteristics[b]	1970.69 (56.9)**	1970.92 (48.8)**
	Differences associated with size, control, and service	
Beds[c]		
Under 100	+1.70 (5.4)**	+1.68 (5.3)**
100–199	Reference class	Reference class
200–299	−0.92 (2.9)**	−0.91 (2.9)**
300 and over	−1.78 (3.6)**	−1.80 (3.7)**
Control		
Private nonprofit	Reference class	Reference class
State and local government	+0.69 (2.0)**	+0.71 (2.0)**
Private, profit	+0.62 (1.7)*	+0.62 (1.7)*
Service		
General	Reference class	Reference class
Specialized	+2.43 (2.9)**	+2.45 (2.9)**
	Differences associated with teaching and research	
Medical school affiliation		
Yes	−1.12 (2.0)**	−1.10 (2.0)**
No	Reference class	Reference class
Residency training program[c]		
Yes	−1.31 (3.7)**	−1.32 (3.7)**
No	Reference class	Reference class
Research grants to hospitals, dollars per bed		
0	Reference class	Reference class
1–99	−0.62 (1.4)	−0.59 (1.3)
100–999	−0.94 (2.0)**	−0.87 (1.7)*
1,000 and over	−1.14 (2.2)**	−1.21 (2.2)**
	Differences associated with patient care	
Doctors per 1,000 beds		
Under 175	+0.01 (0.0)	+0.02 (0.0)
175–249	Reference class	Reference class
250 and over	−0.30 (0.9)	−0.27 (0.8)
Population per bed		
Under 200	−0.17 (0.4)	−0.09 (0.2)
200–249	Reference class	Reference class
250–299	−0.06 (0.2)	−0.05 (0.1)
300 and over	−1.35 (2.6)**	−1.33 (2.5)**
	Differences associated with market structure	
Percent of beds in four largest hospitals		
Under 50	Reference class	Reference class
50–79	+0.39 (1.0)	+0.39 (1.0)
80–100	+0.17 (0.3)	+0.23 (0.4)
Market with fewer than four hospitals	−1.10 (1.6)	−1.05 (1.5)

Table 4-4 (*continued*)

Characteristic	Year	
	Regression excluding third party payment	*Regression including third party payment*
	Differences associated with market structure (*continued*)	
Percent growth in population, 1950–70		
Under 35	Reference class	Reference class
35–59	−0.42 (1.2)	−0.42 (1.2)
60 and over	−0.31 (0.8)	−0.27 (0.6)
Percent of hospitals with diagnostic radioisotopes in 1961		
Under 20	−1.37 (2.9)**	−1.39 (2.9)**
20–39	Reference class	Reference class
40–49	−0.41 (1.2)	−0.53 (1.4)
50 and over	+0.04 (0.1)	−0.09 (0.2)
	Differences associated with third party payment	
Percent of population with hospital insurance, 1963		
Under 65	...	−0.09 (0.1)
65–74	...	+0.13 (0.2)
75–84	...	−0.38 (0.7)
85 and over	...	Reference class
Percent growth in hospital insurance, 1961–71		
Under 10	...	−0.27 (0.4)
10–19	...	Reference class
20–29	...	−0.38 (0.7)
30 and over	...	−0.45 (0.8)
	Differences associated with regulation	
Effective year, certificate-of-need law		
1965–69	+0.70 (1.4)	+0.69 (1.1)
1970–73	+0.31 (1.0)	+0.44 (1.1)
1974–75 or no law	Reference class	Reference class
Summary statistic		
Number of observations	880	880
R^2	0.215	0.216
Corrected R^2	0.192	0.188
F and degrees of freedom [numerator, denominator]	8.98 [26, 853]	7.31 [32, 847]

Sources: See chapter 2 for discussion of the basic data.

* The difference is statistically significant at the 90 percent level of confidence or better, but less than the 95 percent level.

** The difference is statistically significant at the 95 percent level of confidence or better.

a. The numbers in parentheses are *t*-statistics.

b. This is the constant term of the regression and shows the estimated year of adoption for hospitals having all the reference characteristics. (See text for explanation of notion of a reference class.) The values of the dependent variable used in the regressions ranged from 22 (for 1962) to 35 (for 1975), but the constant is expressed here in terms of the corresponding calendar year to make its interpretation more obvious. The *t*-statistic in this case applies not to the number shown but to the difference between that number and 1940 (to 1970.69 − 1940 = 30.69 in column 1, for example).

c. In the year diagnostic radioisotopes were adopted, or, if not available, the year before or after.

Table 4-5. The Year in Which Electroencephalography Was Adopted by a Hospital, 1961–75: Differences Associated with Selected Characteristics of the Hospital and Its Market[a]

	Year	
Characteristic	Regression excluding third party payment	Regression including third party payment
Year for hospitals with all the reference characteristics[b]	1970.50 (56.3)**	1970.41 (51.2)**
	Differences associated with size, control, and service	
Beds[c]		
Under 100	+1.12 (3.0)**	+1.10 (3.0)**
100–199	Reference class	Reference class
200–299	−0.74 (2.4)**	−0.73 (2.4)**
300 and over	−0.86 (2.3)**	−0.83 (2.2)**
Control		
Private nonprofit	Reference class	Reference class
State and local government	+0.26 (0.8)	+0.25 (0.7)
Private, profit	−0.49 (1.2)	−0.41 (1.0)
Service		
General	Reference class	Reference class
Specialized	−0.11 (0.1)	−0.02 (0.0)
	Differences associated with teaching and research	
Medical school affiliation		
Yes	−0.18 (0.4)	−0.25 (0.6)
No	Reference class	Reference class
Residency training program[c]		
Yes	−1.48 (4.8)**	−1.49 (4.8)**
No	Reference class	Reference class
Research grants to hospitals, dollars per bed		
0	Reference class	Reference class
1–99	+0.13 (0.3)	+0.01 (0.0)
100–999	+0.13 (0.3)	−0.06 (0.1)
1,000 and over	−0.69 (1.4)	−0.81 (1.6)
	Differences associated with patient care	
Doctors per 1,000 beds		
Under 175	−0.34 (0.9)	−0.34 (0.9)
175–249	Reference class	Reference class
250 and over	−0.06 (0.2)	+0.03 (0.1)
Percent of beds in intensive care		
0	+0.34 (0.8)	+0.31 (0.7)
Under 4.0	+0.30 (0.9)	+0.26 (0.8)
4.0–5.9	Reference class	Reference class
6.0 and over	+0.25 (0.9)	+0.27 (0.9)
	Differences associated with market structure	
Percent of beds in four largest hospitals		
Under 50	Reference class	Reference class
50–79	+0.36 (1.0)	+0.41 (1.2)
80–100	+0.14 (0.3)	+0.01 (0.0)
Market with fewer than four hospitals	+0.32 (0.5)	+0.12 (0.2)

Table 4-5 (*continued*)

	Year	
Characteristic	*Regression excluding third party payment*	*Regression including third party payment*
	Differences associated with market structure (continued)	
Percent growth in population, 1950–70		
Under 35	Reference class	Reference class
35–59	−0.61 (1.9)*	−0.72 (2.2)**
60 and over	−0.68 (1.9)*	−0.69 (1.8)*
Percent of hospitals with electroencephalograph in 1961		
0	−0.02 (0.0)	+0.12 (0.3)
1–29	Reference class	Reference class
30–44	−0.63 (2.0)**	−0.47 (1.4)
45 and over	−1.01 (2.5)**	−0.97 (2.3)**
	Differences associated with third party payment	
Percent of population with hospital insurance, 1963		
Under 65	...	+1.09 (1.6)
65–74	...	+0.90 (1.5)
75–84	...	+0.63 (1.3)
85 and over	...	Reference class
Percent growth in hospital insurance, 1961–71		
Under 10	...	+0.37 (0.6)
10–19	...	Reference class
20–29	...	−0.85 (1.8)*
30 and over	...	−0.80 (1.5)
	Differences associated with regulation	
Effective year, certificate-of-need law		
1965–69	+0.30 (0.6)	+0.18 (0.3)
1970–73	+0.05 (0.2)	−0.12 (0.3)
1974–75 or no law	Reference class	Reference class
Summary statistic		
Number of observations	1,006	1,006
R^2	0.116	0.122
Corrected R^2	0.094	0.094
F and degrees of freedom [numerator, denominator]	4.96 [26, 979]	4.21 [32, 973]

Sources: See chapter 2 for discussion of the basic data.

* The difference is statistically significant at the 90 percent level of confidence or better, but less than the 95 percent level.

** The difference is statistically significant at the 95 percent level of confidence or better.

a. The numbers in parentheses are *t*-statistics.

b. This is the constant term of the regression and shows the estimated year of adoption for hospitals having all the reference characteristics. (See text for explanation of the notion of a reference class.) The values of the dependent variable used in the regressions ranged from 22 (for 1962) to 35 (for 1975), but the constant is expressed here in terms of the corresponding calendar year to make its interpretation more obvious. The *t*-statistic in this case applies not to the number shown but to the difference between that number and 1940 (to 1970.50 − 1940 = 30.50 in column 1, for example).

c. In the year the electroencephalograph was adopted, or, if not available, the year before or after.

and a half years. It should be noted that these differences probably under-state those that would appear if more early adopters, which tend to be large hospitals, were included in the samples.

The effects of control and type of service differ with the technology. State and local hospitals and specialized hospitals were somewhat slower to adopt respiratory therapy than were private nonprofit and general hospitals, but profit hospitals were not. All three differences were impor-tant for diagnostic radioisotopes: state and local hospitals and profit hos-pitals were moderately slower than nonprofits, and specialized hospitals were slower than general ones by about two and a half years. This last result can probably be explained by the fact that such specialized institu-tions as maternity or rehabilitation hospitals have fewer occasions to test for the kinds of conditions radioisotopes can detect. The electroencephal-ograph was adopted about equally quickly by all hospitals, regardless of control or service.

The estimates for research and teaching also follow the special nature of the technology. Diagnostic radioisotopes are unquestionably the most scientifically prestigious and probably the most scientifically promising of the three. This status shows up in the fact that, while all three technologies were adopted more quickly by hospitals with residency programs, only radioisotopes were influenced by medical school affiliation and research. The estimates are quite large. Medical school affiliation cut the time by more than a year and a commitment to research cut it still further, with the largest programs speeding adoption by another year. Altogether, a large (300 beds or more) medical center hospital in an area that received the highest level of research funds adopted diagnostic radioisotopes more than five years earlier than did the reference group hospitals—in 1965 rather than 1970 (from the first column, $1970.69 - 1.78 - 1.12 - 1.31 - 1.14 = 1965.34$).

In general, the factors listed under patient care show little effect on the speed of diffusion. None of the technologies was influenced by the number of doctors in the area; the specialty distribution was also unim-portant.[51] Deaths from respiratory disease are not related to hospitals' decisions to adopt respiratory therapy nor, in spite of the importance of the EEG in the intensive care unit, is the percent of the hospital's beds

51. Diagnostic radioisotopes and respiratory therapy showed a tendency to be adopted more readily where there were fewer general practitioners. The EEG showed a less easily explained tendency to be adopted more quickly where there were fewer doctors in the medical specialties.

allocated to intensive care in 1975 related to that technology's adoption.[52] But population per hospital bed (a proxy for the incidence of more specific conditions) does help to explain the diffusion of diagnostic radioisotopes; hospitals in areas with 300 or more people per bed adopted this technology 1.3 years sooner than hospitals in other areas.

As in the last chapter, the degree of concentration in the market shows no systematic or significant relationship with the speed of diffusion. The growth of population was important for the electroencephalograph: hospitals in areas where that growth exceeded 35 percent over the two decades between 1950 and 1970 adopted it about eight months sooner than other hospitals. It played no part in the diffusion of the other two technologies.[53]

The stimulus of example also played a part in the adoption of the EEG. Hospitals in areas where 30 percent to 44 percent of the hospitals had already adopted it by 1961 subsequently introduced it about six months sooner, and where the level in 1961 exceeded 45 percent, the remaining hospitals adopted a full year sooner. The pattern for the adoption of diagnostic radioisotopes is a rather curious one, at variance both with the results for the EEG and with the analysis of intensive care in chapter 3. Possibly it reflects a situation in which certain hospitals responded to the influence of regional or national leaders rather than local ones in adopting this prestigious technology; but this hypothesis is difficult to test and was not tested.

For the most part, the results for third party payment are statistically insignificant, although, as before, the quality of the data prohibit drawing any firm conclusions from this outcome. There is, however, an interesting exception. For the electroencephalograph, the pattern of differences is what one would have predicted: adoption was slower in areas where the level of hospital insurance was lower, and the estimated delay declines in stair-step fashion as the level of insurance rises; further, adoption was faster in areas where the growth of insurance was faster. Only one of the

52. The year in which the hospital adopted intensive care was also tried and was significantly related to the adoption of the EEG. But it seemed likely that this simply represented a tendency on the part of the hospital to adopt all technologies early—a hypothesis that was supported by the fact that the number of beds was reduced to insignificance in these regressions—rather than any special connection between intensive care and the EEG.

53. The lack of an effect on diagnostic radioisotopes is not due to the inclusion of population per bed in those regressions. The results were the same in specifications that omitted population per bed.

six estimates is significant at the 90 percent level, but four more are significant at the 80 percent level. These results are particularly intriguing because they are matched in the next chapter by the results for cobalt therapy. Both of these technologies were introduced to a greater degree in the 1950s and early 1960s than were any of the others considered in the study. A plausible hypothesis is that differences between areas in insurance coverage mattered when there was less of it but that at the high levels of more recent years the remaining differences are unimportant.

For the reasons discussed in chapter 3 in connection with the analysis of the adoption of intensive care units, the only regulatory measure that could be tested for all three technologies was certificate-of-need laws. The regional medical and comprehensive health planning programs were tested for respiratory therapy, since all the hospitals in the sample introduced it after the starting dates of these programs; the lack of significant results, while plausible enough, cannot be given much weight, since the analysis is based on such a narrow segment of the diffusion process. The lack of any effect for certificate-of-need laws is, however, repeated across all three technologies: none of them has been slowed in its diffusion by certificate-of-need reviews.[54] Some certificate-of-need laws require review only of proposed investments that exceed a certain dollar limit. All three of these technologies can be introduced at relatively low cost, and it is possible that many review boards had no chance to influence them because they seldom qualified for review.

Overall, the results of these analyses agree in many instances with the results of chapter 3, especially those for the parallel analysis of the speed of diffusion of intensive care. Certain patterns have now been repeated several times and begin to point to general influences on the diffusion of medical technologies, some of which may be amenable to policy intervention. As noted earlier, these common patterns are reviewed in chapter 7, where they can be combined with the results reported in the next chapter.

54. The method used to test certificate-of-need legislation was the same one described in chapter 3. Three classes were defined based on the effective year of the law: 1965–69; 1970–73; and 1974–75 or no law. Hospitals were assigned to the class in which their state law belonged, whether they adopted the technology before or after the law went into effect. The percentages of hospitals that adopted while the law was in effect are, in the same order as the classes: 98 percent, 35 percent, and less than 1 percent for respiratory therapy; 68 percent, 35 percent, and less than 1 percent for diagnostic radioisotopes; and 64 percent, 29 percent, and 4 percent for the electroencephalograph.

chapter five **The Distribution of Prestige Technologies:**
Cobalt Therapy, Open-Heart Surgery, and
Renal Dialysis

The three technologies that are the subject of this chapter—cobalt radiotherapy, open-heart surgery, and renal dialysis—are familiar to most people from newspaper headlines. In its day, each has been publicized as a shining example of the potential of modern medicine and an important advance over what had been possible until then. Cobalt radiotherapy is the oldest of the three and has, in fact, been replaced at the frontier of radiotherapy by other, newer, technologies. Open-heart surgery and renal dialysis are somewhat more recent and are still very much in the news, although the articles now tend to deal with matters like overuse and high costs rather than with the excitement of their early promise.

All three share certain common characteristics. Each depends on impressively complex equipment: the cobalt teletherapy unit, which focuses the radioactivity produced spontaneously by cobalt; the heart-lung machine, which can temporarily take over the functions of the human circulatory system; and the artificial kidney. Each requires specially and often highly trained staff and an array of supporting facilities such as diagnostic laboratories, radiophysics laboratories, and intensive care units—not all of them necessarily in the hospital itself, but close enough for consultation. Each serves a sharply defined—and in the cases of open-heart surgery and renal dialysis, numerically small—group of patients. Part of the reason for the sharp boundaries is that these technologies involve much higher risks of death and injury than do the more common hospital services.

For all of these reasons, all three technologies are concentrated in large hospitals (figure 5-1). Very few hospitals of less than 200 beds have them,

Figure 5-1. Percent of Nonfederal Short-Term Hospitals with Cobalt Therapy, Open-Heart Surgery, and Renal Dialysis, by Size of Hospital, 1976

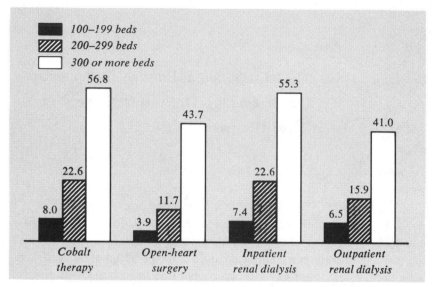

Source: *Hospital Statistics, 1977 Edition: Data from the American Hospital Association 1976 Annual Survey*, table 12A.

and even among hospitals of 200 to 299 beds, those reporting the technologies are in a definite minority. For each of the three technologies, the period of rapid diffusion had ended by the late 1960s—earlier for cobalt —and the proportions in the chart represent the final plateau of adoption, or something close to it.

The regional distribution of the technologies, shown in table 5-1, gives an indication of their availability to the population in different parts of the country. Ratios of facilities to population are, of course, only a rough indicator of availability, since the regions cover such different land areas: four units per one million population may represent longer average driving times in one area than three units per million represents in a more densely populated area. And in the case of outpatient dialysis, while the number of hospital units per million gives some idea of geographic accessibility, it says nothing about the capacity of those units (the numbers of dialysis stations per million would be a much better measure), and it ignores the fact that a sizable number of dialysis centers are not associated with hospitals; of the 840 centers approved for Medicare reimbursement in 1977, 190 were nonhospital facilities. For cobalt, open-heart surgery, and inpatient dialysis, the unit—its existence or nonexistence—is an imperfect but much more reasonable indicator of capacity.

The ratios show that no one region is always the worst off. The South Atlantic has the fewest cobalt units relative to its population, but New England has the fewest open-heart surgery units, and the East South Central region the fewest dialysis facilities. Further, the ratio of beds to population—a measure often used to compare the hospital resources of different areas—does not accurately reflect the availability of more specific kinds of hospital resources: the Mountain states have fewer beds per thousand than the national average but more open-heart surgery and dialysis units.

In the case of cobalt therapy, the equipment ratios prescribed by the French Ministry of Health for the regions of that country (see chapter 6) provide the basis for a rather interesting comparison. The first ratio, published in 1973, set five cobalt units per million population as the desirable number. Not one of the nine regions in table 5-1 had reached that ratio in 1976.[1]

The rest of this chapter is divided into two parts. The first part presents brief accounts of each of the three technologies. The second part of the chapter presents the statistical analysis of the distribution of these technologies among hospitals. Since the American Hospital Association survey missed the years during which they spread, it is not possible to analyze the speed of their adoption. Instead the analysis investigates the factors that have influenced the level of adoption finally reached, as represented by the level in 1975.

Cobalt Therapy[2]

Radiation therapy is used almost exclusively for the treatment of cancer: to cure it or, when that is not possible, to alleviate its symptoms.

1. The French recently changed the regulation so that both cobalt therapy units and linear accelerators of less than 10 million volts are counted toward the ratio of five per million. There are no separate data for the United States on these accelerators (they are lumped together with other types of X-ray therapy in the American Hospital Association's statistics), so that it is impossible to tell how the regions of the United States would fare against the new standard.

2. For a somewhat more detailed case study of radiotherapy, see Louise B. Russell, "The Diffusion of New Hospital Technologies in the United States," *International Journal of Health Services*, vol. 6, no. 4 (1976), pp. 557–80 (Brookings Reprint 322).

Table 5-1. Regional Distributions of Cobalt Therapy, Open-Heart Surgery, and Renal Dialysis Units, and of Hospital Beds, 1976[a]

Region	Cobalt therapy units		Open-heart surgery units		Inpatient dialysis units		Outpatient dialysis units		
	Total	Per million population	Total	Per million population	Total	Per million population	Total	Per million population	Beds per thousand population
New England	43	3.52	21	1.72	49	4.01	36	2.95	4.53
Middle Atlantic	156	4.18	76	2.04	152	4.08	123	3.30	4.94
South Atlantic	104	3.06	84	2.47	146	4.30	94	2.77	4.86
East North Central	182	4.45	104	2.54	139	3.40	124	3.03	5.04
East South Central	56	4.10	30	2.20	35	2.56	32	2.34	5.34
West North Central	76	4.52	50	2.98	59	3.51	63	3.75	6.30
West South Central	82	3.87	83	3.91	99	4.67	76	3.58	5.16
Mountain	32	3.25	36	3.66	49	4.98	39	3.97	4.43
Pacific	106	3.69	102	3.55	145	5.05	106	3.69	4.24
United States	837	3.90	586	2.73	873	4.07	693	3.23	4.96

Sources: Units and beds, *Hospital Statistics, 1977 Edition: Data from the American Hospital Association 1976 Annual Survey*, tables 5B, 12B; population, U.S. Bureau of the Census, *Current Population Reports*, series P-25, no. 642, "Revised 1975 and Provisional 1976 Estimates of the Population of States, and Components of Change, 1970 to 1976" (Government Printing Office, 1976), table 1.

a. Number of units and beds in "federal general and other special" plus "nonfederal short-term general and other special" hospitals.

There are approximately 300 new cases of cancer per 100,000 population each year. Adding previously discovered cases, 430 people per 100,000 receive treatment for cancer during a given year. The proportion who receive radiation therapy at some point during their illness is quite large—about 70 percent—and is fairly equally divided between those for whom radiation is prescribed as a possible cure and those for whom it serves to relieve the side effects of an incurable cancer.[3]

Radiation therapy is seldom used alone in the treatment of cancer. For many of the major cancers—cancers of the lung, breast, bladder, and ovaries, for example—surgery is the primary method of therapy and radiation is used as a supplement, to try to kill any cancerous tissue that might have been missed by the surgery. For some cancers, radiation is combined with chemotherapy. And for still others, all three therapies are used.

The difficulty with all three forms of treatment is that their effects are not specific to cancer. They damage normal tissue as well. Over the years, this problem has stimulated constant experimentation aimed at mini-

3. Franz Buschke and Robert G. Parker, *Radiation Therapy in Cancer Management* (Grune and Stratton, 1972), p. 4; Ned B. Hornback, L. E. Cloe, and David J. Edwards, "Report of Radiation Therapy and Therapeutic Radioisotope Facilities and Personnel in Indiana: A Model for Projecting Need in 1980," *Journal of the Indiana State Medical Association*, vol. 69 (July 1976), pp. 508–09. Although radiotherapy is a hospital-based technology, most patients do not need to be hospitalized but are treated as outpatients.

mizing side effects and focusing therapy more sharply on the cancer by the use of new methods, new combinations of therapies, and new ways of increasing the sensitivity of the cancer to therapy. In radiotherapy this experimentation has involved the investigation of different types and strengths of radioactivity. While the biological effects of all forms of radiation are thought to be essentially the same,[4] radioactive sources vary considerably in the way their rays are absorbed by the body, so that each offers the possibility of some unique advantage for certain kinds of cancer.

Cobalt achieved its importance as a teletherapy source (in teletherapy, radiation is beamed at the patient from a source outside his body) because it was the first good, relatively inexpensive, source of supervoltage quality. The quality, or penetrating power, of radiation is measured in thousands of volts (kilovolts) or millions of volts, and teletherapy sources are conventionally distinguished as orthovoltage (less than one million volts) or supervoltage (one million volts or more), or, more recently, megavoltage (ten to twelve million volts or more). Orthovoltage sources deliver their maximum dose to the skin and are thus best for treating cancers on or very close to the surface. As the penetrating power of the source increases into the supervoltage range, several important changes take place.[5] The higher the voltage, the farther below the surface it delivers its maximum dose and the lower the proportion of that dose delivered to the skin. This means that a much larger dose can be delivered to deep tumors before the skin reaction calls a halt to further treatment. Supervoltage is also better focused than orthovoltage, so that less is scattered to normal tissues surrounding the tumor and less is absorbed by the bones. And compared to an earlier supervoltage source, radium, cobalt is not only less expensive and better focused but safer; like all spontaneously radioactive sources, radium decays, but unlike cobalt it produces a radioactive gas as it does so, which builds up pressure on its container and creates a potential for radioactive spills.

Once a practical unit was developed in the early 1950s, cobalt became the accepted form of radiation therapy for many of the major cancers,

4. Buschke and Parker, *Radiation Therapy in Cancer Management,* chap. 3; Ronald E. Waggener, "Radiotherapy Terms and Tools," *Nebraska State Medical Journal,* vol. 52 (December 1967), pp. 526–29.

5. Buschke and Parker, *Radiation Therapy in Cancer Management,* chap. 3; Gilbert H. Fletcher, "Supervoltage Roentgentherapy: Clinical Evaluation Based on 2,000 Cases," *Texas State Journal of Medicine,* vol. 55 (August 1959), pp. 676–78; John D. Watson, Jr., and William S. Maxfield, "Cobalt Therapy: When and Why," *Journal of the Louisiana State Medical Society,* vol. 119 (July 1967), pp. 272–77.

Figure 5-2. Percent of Private Nonprofit Hospitals with 200 through 299 Beds Reporting Selected Radiotherapy Facilities, 1960–76[a]

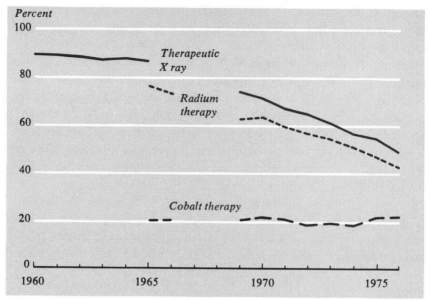

Sources: *Hospitals, Journal of the American Hospital Association*, vol. 45 (August 1, 1971), Guide Issue, pt. 2, and preceding annual guide issues; and *Hospital Statistics*, annual issues.
a. Gaps in the lines reflect years in which the facility was omitted from the survey.

displacing orthovoltage X-ray and radium (see figure 5-2). As these things go, it is still relatively inexpensive and easy to maintain. In 1975 the total cost of a cobalt teletherapy unit ranged from $90,000 to $125,000. Maintenance is fairly simple because the radiation is spontaneously produced, but by the same token the source decays steadily—over a half-life of 5.3 years—and must be replaced at regular intervals; recommendations range from every three to every eight years.[6]

But the history of radiotherapy is a succession of competing technologies, and cobalt's position has been repeatedly challenged by other types of radioactivity. In the 1960s there was considerable interest in the potential of the electron beam, because the dose delivered by an electron beam drops off sharply after it reaches a certain depth, with obvious ad-

6. T. Ashton and A. E. Chester, "The Economics of High-Intensity Cobalt 60 Therapy Sources," *British Journal of Radiology*, vol. 35 (October 1962), pp. 704–09; M. Lederman, "Advances in Radiotherapy," *Practitioner*, vol. 205 (October 1970), pp. 535–43.

vantages for cases in which it is important to minimize the radiation of normal structures that lie beyond the tumor.[7] This advantage must be weighed against the poor focus of the beam, which scatters radiation to normal tissue around the cancer. High-energy x-radiation produced by linear accelerators in the megavoltage range has also taken part of the field away from cobalt.[8] It offers further improvements in dose patterns along the lines of those supervoltage has over orthovoltage, although the magnitude of these advantages is apparently considerably less (Buschke and Parker refer to megavoltage sources as "a tidbit for the radiologic gourmet").[9] As a third example, fast neutrons have attracted attention in this decade because they are more effective with poorly oxygenated cells and it is known that some tumor cells are poorly oxygenated.[10] Like the electron beam, fast neutrons suffer from relatively poor focus, but cyclotrons designed for medical use are nonetheless being installed in a few hospitals around the world.[11]

Rather than eliminating older types of radiotherapy, each new source increases the range of equipment considered necessary for a good radiotherapy center and narrows the field of application of each source. One advisory committee recommended recently that a fully equipped center, with no pretensions to being a special educational facility or a research facility, should have both a supervoltage and a megavoltage source as well as orthovoltage and superficial (about fifty kilovolts) machines.[12] The cost of all this equipment is considerable. One recently built center

7. Norah duV. Tapley, "The Electron Beam in Tumor Therapy," *Hospital Practice*, vol. 3 (June 1968), pp. 48–51.

8. An electron beam is usually provided as an option on linear accelerators in this range.

9. *Radiation Therapy in Cancer Management*, p. 18.

10. G. W. Barendsen, "Characteristics of Tumour Responses to Different Radiations and the Relative Biological Effectiveness of Fast Neutrons," *European Journal of Cancer*, vol. 10 (May 1974), pp. 269–74; K. Breur, "International Cooperation with Regard to Clinical Trials of Fast Neutron Radiotherapy," ibid., vol. 10 (June 1974), pp. 385–86; W. Duncan, "Fast Neutron Therapy: Past and Present," *Acta Rad'ologica*, vol. 313, Supplement (1972), pp. 11–32; H.-J. Eichhorn, A. Lessel, and S. Matschke, "Comparison between Neutron Therapy and ^{60}Co Gamma Ray Therapy of Bronchial, Gastric and Oesophagus Carcinomata," *European Journal of Cancer*, vol. 10 (June 1974), pp. 361–64.

11. "New Machine for Cancer Patients," *Hospital International* [London] vol. 10 (August 1976), pp. 3–4.

12. Hornback and others, "Report of Radiation Therapy and Therapeutic Radioisotope Facilities and Personnel in Indiana."

spent over a million dollars to acquire two cobalt units, a linear accelerator, an orthovoltage unit, and supporting equipment.[13] Construction costs are also high because of the need to shield staff, and the surrounding population, from stray radiation.

It is difficult to evaluate the benefits of radiation therapy. The question is complicated not only by the fact that radiation is generally used in combination with other therapies, but by the fact that its benefits—which are often those of short-term palliation rather than cure—must be weighed against its sometimes serious side effects. If it is difficult to evaluate the benefits of radiation therapy in general, it is even more difficult to say anything about the benefits of particular new forms of radiation. But given the lack of significant improvement in the mortality rates for most cancers since the 1950s,[14] it seems safe to conclude that the search for the perfect form of radiation for each cancer is another case in which large investments are being made in return for small benefits.

Open-Heart Surgery

Surgery directly on the exposed heart moved out of the category of a medical curiosity with the development of the pump-oxygenator, or heart-lung machine—a machine that can temporarily take over the job of the heart and lungs—in the 1950s. Once the pump-oxygenator was available, surgeons began to perfect various procedures to repair or replace defective parts of the heart. The procedures in common use today include the surgical repair of the valves and walls of the heart, the replacement of natural heart valves with man-made ones, and the best-known procedure of all, the bypass graft, in which portions of the blood vessels leading into or out of the heart, which have become partially blocked because of arteriosclerosis, are replaced with lengths of blood vessel taken from elsewhere in the patient's body.

The bypass graft has been the major element in the rapid growth of open-heart procedures. In 1967, about 14,000 procedures of all kinds

13. Maria R. Traska, "St. Joseph's Builds Oncology Center Underground: Cuts Construction Costs," *Modern Healthcare: Short-term Care Edition,* vol. 6 (December 1976), pp. 42–43.

14. Sidney J. Cutler, Max H. Myers, and Sylvan B. Green, "Trends in Survival Rates of Patients with Cancer," *New England Journal of Medicine,* vol. 293 (July 17, 1975), pp. 122–24.

Figure 5-3. Percent of Hospitals with Open-Heart Surgery Units, by Size of Hospital and Type of Control, 1969–76

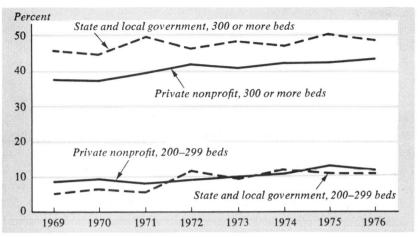

Sources: Same as figure 5-2.

were performed. By 1971, only four years later, the number had grown to more than 38,000, and today it is estimated that 70,000 bypass graft procedures alone are done each year.[15] This growth appears to have come about through the increased use of existing facilities rather than the introduction of new ones. As figure 5-3 illustrates, the upward trend in the proportions of hospitals reporting open-heart surgery units has been quite gentle, not at all like the trend in the number of procedures.

Open-heart surgery is expensive and even a brief list of the required equipment and support facilities, not to mention the staff to run them, suggests why. In addition to the pump-oxygenator, the other equipment needed in the operating room includes a battery of electronic monitoring devices to chart the patient's condition while the surgery is going on and life support equipment—defibrillators, respirators, and the like—for use in emergencies. Clinical laboratory facilities, particularly for blood-gas analyses, and radiology facilities must be nearby. Open-heart surgery depends on a constellation of technologies outside the operating room as well—a sophisticated radiology department and cardiac catheterization lab for presurgical diagnosis, a blood bank to supply blood during the

15. James K. Roche and James M. Stengle, "Facilities for Open Heart Surgery in the United States: Distribution, Utilization and Cost," *American Journal of Cardiology*, vol. 32 (August 1973), pp. 224–28; "Heart Bypasses Are Often Unnecessary, Study Says," *New York Times*, March 10, 1977.

operation, and an intensive care unit to watch over the patient when the surgery is done.[16]

There are no published data for recent years that give the investment costs of these facilities, or even of those parts—like certain operating room equipment, and the cardiac catheterization lab—that are specific to open-heart surgery. There are, however, some rather rough estimates of the charge for an operation. These put the cost of a single procedure at $10,000 to $15,000.[17] Both estimates include the hospital charges connected with the surgery, and the higher one appears to include physicians' fees. Neither includes the charges for diagnosis, which may take place some time before the admission for surgery.

Only a few years ago the concern most often voiced about open-heart surgery units was that expensive equipment was being underused—there were too many units for the number of operations being done. A survey conducted by the National Institutes of Health found that 62 percent of the hospitals in the United States with open-heart surgery units reported fewer than 100 operations performed during 1971.[18] At that time the Surgery Study Group of the Inter-Society Commission for Heart Disease Resources was recommending 200 operations per year as the minimum necessary to maintain the skills of the surgical team, and in Britain the Joint Cardiology Committee of the Royal Colleges of Physicians and Surgeons had recommended an annual workload of about 300 open-heart procedures as necessary to make good use of the capital investment.[19]

As the popularity of the surgery has grown and experience with it has accumulated the questions have become instead, What are its benefits, and for which kinds of patients? The questioning has been directed primarily at the bypass graft procedure. This procedure is now being performed on patients who have only mild symptoms, or no overt symptoms

16. Louise B. Russell and Carol S. Burke, *Technological Diffusion in the Hospital Sector,* prepared for the National Science Foundation (National Planning Association, October 1975; available from the National Technical Information Service, report no. PB 245 642/AS), chap. 5.

17. Eldred D. Mundth and W. Gerald Austen, "Surgical Measures for Coronary Heart Disease," *New England Journal of Medicine,* vol. 293 (July 3, 1975), pp. 13–19; ibid. (July 10, 1975), pp. 75–80; ibid. (July 17, 1975), pp. 124–30; "Heart Bypasses Are Often Unnecessary," *New York Times,* March 10, 1977.

18. Roche and Stengle, "Facilities for Open Heart Surgery," p. 226.

19. Roche and Stengle, "Facilities for Open Heart Surgery"; "A Combined Medical and Surgical Unit for Cardiac Surgery," Report of the Joint Cardiology Committee of the Royal Colleges of Physicians and Surgeons, *British Heart Journal,* vol. 30 (November 1968), pp. 864–68.

at all (one physician estimates that as many as 25 percent of the current number of operations is for these patients)[20] because it is widely believed that it reduces the chance of death from heart attack. For the most part, this belief is untested.

A spate of studies on various aspects of the issue has been published in the last few years.[21] It is generally agreed that surgery is more successful than medical treatment at relieving the pain of angina pectoris (a condition characterized by sharp, constricting, chest pains and often caused by partially blocked arteries). It is apparently also accepted that surgery improves the chances of survival for patients who have main left coronary artery disease and stable angina (the main left artery supplies the left ventricle of the heart with oxygen). It might be possible to get agreement that surgery is not a good idea when the patient has only one diseased vessel, and that one is not the main left artery, but here the consensus begins to disintegrate.

The early results from a study of the bypass graft procedure conducted by the Veterans Administration have generated a great deal of interest and argument.[22] One of the reasons is that, unlike its predecessors, this study assigned patients randomly to either medical therapy or surgery, so that patient selection could not bias the outcome. And since it already had been shown that patients with main left artery disease experience lower mortality when they are treated surgically rather than medically, patients with this condition were excluded from the study altogether. The results show that, after three years, the mortality rates of the surgically and medically treated groups were virtually identical—13 percent for the medically treated group, 12 percent for the surgically treated group. When the two groups were subdivided by the extent of heart disease, and matching subgroups were compared, there were still no differences. In this first report, the authors did not evaluate the effectiveness of surgery in relieving pain.

20. Lawrence Meyer, "Heart Operation Called Questionable," *Washington Post,* July 26, 1977.

21. Karl E. Hammermeister and others, "Effect of Aortocoronary Saphenous Vein Bypass Grafting on Death and Sudden Death," *American Journal of Cardiology,* vol. 39 (May 26, 1977), pp. 925–34; Marvin L. Murphy and others, "Treatment of Chronic Stable Angina: A Preliminary Report of Survival Data of the Randomized Veterans Administration Cooperative Study," *New England Journal of Medicine,* vol. 297 (September 22, 1977), pp. 621–27; Albert Oberman and others, "Surgical versus Medical Treatment in Disease of the Left Main Coronary Artery," *Lancet,* vol. 2, no. 7986 (September 18, 1976), pp. 591–94.

22. Murphy and others, "Treatment of Chronic Stable Angina."

Many people feel strongly about the issue and this article in particular has provoked a great deal of controversy. In a departure from its usual policy, the *New England Journal* devoted several pages of the issue of December 29, 1977, to the letters that inundated the editors after the article appeared. The study is not the first, although it is probably the most persuasive, to suggest that the use of open-heart surgery is being pushed to the point of negligible benefit. The sequence of events is unfortunately a common one: the growth of the technology preceded testing and will undoubtedly continue during the controversy over the early test results.

Renal Dialysis[23]

An artificial kidney filters metabolic wastes from the blood in essentially the same fashion as a natural kidney.[24] In all of the different types of artificial kidney the patient's blood is allowed to flow along one side of a semipermeable membrane—a membrane through which molecules of less than a certain size can pass, but larger molecules cannot—while dialysis solution flows along the other. The major waste products are small enough to move through the membrane, passing from the blood into the dialysis fluid until the concentrations on both sides of the membrane are equal. Protein molecules and blood cells are too large to pass through the membrane and remain in the blood to be carried back into the patient.

The basic principles of dialysis have been understood for a long time. The first dialysis machine was invented in 1913 and the first practical machine in 1943.[25] For a number of years dialysis was used to a limited extent in the treatment of acute renal failure, where one or a few dialyses are enough to keep the patient going until his own kidney can function normally again. But it was not until dialysis could be used for patients with chronic kidney disease—those whose kidneys have deteriorated to

23. A more detailed case study of renal dialysis is available in the report prepared for the National Science Foundation on which this book is based: Louise B. Russell, *Technology in Hospitals: Medical Advances and Their Diffusion* (May 1978), app. D. The full report is available from the National Technical Information Service, report no. PB 287 648/AS; the appendix alone can be obtained from the author on request.

24. The following description is from Joan DeLong Harrington and Etta Rae Brener, *Patient Care in Renal Failure* (Saunders, 1973), pp. 114–16.

25. Ibid., p. 113; John H. Holmgren, "What the Buyer Needs to Know About Dialyzers," *Modern Healthcare: Short-term Care Edition,* vol. 6 (July 1976), pp. 52–53.

the point that they can no longer keep the patient in reasonable health, and death is imminent—that renal dialysis came to assume the prominent place it now holds among medical technologies. This new use was made possible by a series of inventions and experiments in the late 1950s and early 1960s that produced a dialysis machine that was reasonably simple to operate, the first method for creating a permanent entryway into the circulatory system so that dialysis could be repeated frequently, and the experience to show that it was not only possible but beneficial to dialyze people with chronic kidney failure.[26]

The first programs of long-term dialysis were set up in the early 1960s, supported in large part by federal money for medical research and, a little later, federal money for the demonstration of new medical techniques.[27] By 1967 about 1,000 people were on long-term dialysis, but it was estimated that another 6,000 died each year because there was not enough money to treat them. These numbers represent approximately thirty-five new dialysis patients per million population each year.

The number of programs and the number of patients on dialysis continued to grow during the later 1960s and the early 1970s (figures 5-4 and 5-5 chart the growth of the programs).[28] As they grew, the pressure mounted for the federal government to do something to relieve patients and other payers of the expensive burden of this treatment and to make it more widely available. On July 1, 1973, as a result of legislation passed in 1972, the Medicare program began to help pay the costs of dialysis and kidney transplants for virtually anyone who needed them. By June 1977 there were approximately 35,000 dialysis patients receiving Medicare benefits and the number is expected to grow to 60,000 or more by the mid-1980s.[29]

26. Serafino Garella, Joseph A. Chazan, and Sewell I. Kahn, "Treatment of End Stage Renal Disease in Rhode Island: A Status Report," *Rhode Island Medical Journal*, vol. 58 (April 1975), pp. 151–55, 168–69; Harrington and Brener, *Patient Care in Renal Failure*, pp. 113–14.

27. Herbert E. Klarman, John O'S. Francis, and Gerald D. Rosenthal, "Cost Effectiveness Analysis Applied to the Treatment of Chronic Renal Disease," *Medical Care*, vol. 6 (January–February 1968), pp. 48–54.

28. Figure 5-4 shows hospital dialysis programs, which are only part, albeit the largest part, of the total. As of January 1977, 190 of the 840 facilities approved by Medicare were not associated with hospitals.

29. "Quarterly Statistical Summary, Quarter Ending 06/30/77," tabulation provided by U.S. Department of Health, Education, and Welfare, Health Care Financing Administration, Chronic Renal Disease Branch, August 30, 1977; *Medicare End-Stage Renal Disease Program Amendments*, Hearing before the House Committee on Ways and Means, 95 Cong. 1 sess. (Government Printing Office, 1977).

Figure 5-4. Percent of Hospitals with Outpatient Renal Dialysis Facilities, by Size of Hospital and Type of Control, 1968–76

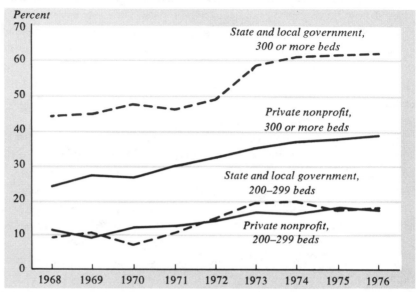

Sources: Same as figure 5-2.

Today the most frequently quoted estimate of new patients is sixty per million per year, compared to thirty-five per million ten years ago.[30] The difference is due to the changes that have taken place in patient selection in response to the more liberal financing. In 1967, when the number of places in dialysis programs was much smaller than the number of people with kidney failure, admissions committees used a number of criteria to help them select those patients for whom the treatment seemed likely to provide the greatest benefit. The Committee on Chronic Kidney Disease recommended that first priority go to patients between fifteen and forty-five years of age and that the patients selected should, except for their kidney disease, be in basically good health—they should not have any other irremediable disease; severe arteriosclerotic heart disease and hypertension were mentioned specifically.[31]

30. Garella and others, "Treatment of End Stage Renal Disease"; Dan B. Mc-Laughlin and Fred L. Shapiro, "Regional Kidney Disease Network Offers Efficient Care, Operation," *Hospitals, Journal of the American Hospital Association,* vol. 50 (January 1, 1976), pp. 89–92; Joseph S. Pliskin and others, "Hemodialysis—Projecting Future Bed Needs: Deterministic and Probabilistic Forecasting," *Computers and Biomedical Research,* vol. 9 (August 1976), p. 319.

31. Klarman and others, "Cost Effectiveness Analysis."

Figure 5-5. Percent of Hospitals with Inpatient Renal Dialysis Facilities, by Size of Hospital and Type of Control, 1968–76

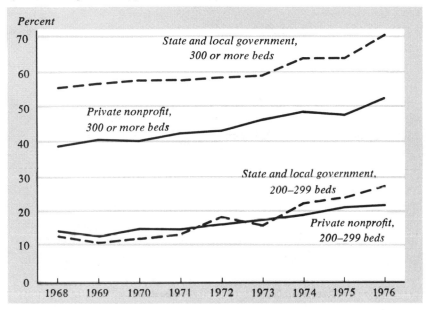

Sources: Same as figure 5-2.

Ten years later there is essentially only one criterion for acceptance into a dialysis program—disabling uremia (uremia is an excess of metabolic wastes in the blood). Very young and very old people are accepted, and a large proportion of dialysis patients suffer from serious diseases other than kidney failure—cancer, diabetes, and liver disease among them.[32] The estimate of sixty new patients per million reflects these more liberal admissions criteria.

Another shift, which started with the introduction of Medicare financing for dialysis and which has caused considerable concern in Congress, is the shift from dialysis at home to dialysis in outpatient centers. Dialysis is provided in a number of settings—inpatient hospital units, outpatient hospital units, freestanding outpatient centers that may or may not be associated with hospitals, and the patient's home. In 1972, just before Medicare started paying for dialysis, 40 percent of all dialysis patients dialyzed at home. In 1977, when Congress reviewed the Medicare pro-

32. Garella and others, "Treatment of End Stage Renal Disease"; Roger Platt, "Planning for Dialysis and Transplantation Facilities," *Medical Care,* vol. 11 (May–June 1973), pp. 199–213.

gram for kidney disease patients, this proportion had dropped to less than 20 percent, although in Europe the proportion had continued to rise over the same years.[33]

The shift is a matter for concern because, as with every other medical care program, the costs of the dialysis program have far outstripped the original estimates. As of June 1977, the costs paid by Medicare ran at an annual rate of $16,800 per patient, even though Medicare does not pay all the costs of dialysis.[34] Home care is, of course, less expensive than dialysis in any other setting. One recent study estimates that in 1973 the costs of dialysis were $6,729 per year at home, $16,520 per year in a limited-care outpatient center, and $24,738 per year in a hospital out-patient center.[35]

These estimates were carefully prepared in order to maintain comparability, but they are not complete. They exclude the costs of radiology, physicians' services, and the surgery necessary to create the permanent entryway into the patient's circulatory system. Perhaps most important, they ignore the fact that the different settings are not mutually exclusive in practice. An estimate is given for the costs of dialysis during the training period that home dialysis patients must go through, but no attempt is made to estimate the costs that result when home or center patients must be admitted to the hospital because of problems with the dialysis, or for treatment of the complications of the disease itself, or when home patients must return to a center. Thus the data give only a rough indication of the actual cost differences associated with different settings.

The trends in renal dialysis are consistent with the results one would expect in response to a financing program aimed at removing costs as a constraint. Renal dialysis is clearly of benefit to the patient. While it is not without risks, it unquestionably prolongs the lives of people who would be unable to survive without it. Quite naturally, as the costs to the people making the decisions have declined, the procedure has been extended to people who gain less from it in terms of added years or months of life and of the quality of that life. And, increasingly, dialysis is being done in outpatient centers, where it costs more than at home. Heated arguments arise over whether the benefits of the switch from home to center accrue to

33. *Medicare End-Stage Renal Disease Program Amendments,* p. 73.
34. "Quarterly Statistical Summary, Quarter ending 06/30/77."
35. Paul A. Hoffstein, Keatha K. Krueger, and Robert J. Wineman, "Dialysis Costs: Results of A Diverse Sample Study," *Kidney International,* vol. 9 (March 1976), pp. 286–93.

the patient, but it appears to be a question on which honest people can differ. Nonetheless, one can accept that there may be such benefits without losing sight of the fact that they are small relative to the cost. The shift to centers is consistent with the more general tendency to push investment to the point of small or zero benefit when the costs facing those who make the decisions are small or zero.

The Statistical Analysis

The analysis presented in this section is based on the 2,772 hospitals that were located in metropolitan areas in 1975 and responded to the American Hospital Association survey in that year—the same hospitals used for the analysis of intensive care beds. Some of the characteristics of these hospitals, including their distribution by number of beds, are described in chapter 2. With respect to the technologies of interest for this chapter, 23.3 percent of the hospitals reported cobalt therapy in 1975 and 17.9 percent reported open-heart surgery units. Somewhat more (22.7 percent) reported inpatient dialysis—which often means no more than the ability to provide a few treatments to critically ill patients—than outpatient dialysis (17.3 percent).

The results of the analysis are presented in tables 5-2, 5-3, and 5-4. As in the preceding chapters, the potential explanatory factors are listed down the left side of each table.[36] Table 5-2 shows two regressions for cobalt therapy; data representing third party payment are excluded from the regression in the first column and included in the one in the second column. Similarly, table 5-3 gives two regressions explaining open-heart surgery units, one with and one without third party payment. Table 5-4 presents one regression each for inpatient renal dialysis (first column) and outpatient renal dialysis (second column). The analysis of this technology was less successful than the analyses of the other two, in terms of the number of factors that were statistically significant and the plausibility and interest of the results, and it did not seem to add anything to present the results two ways. For the same reasons, the results for renal dialysis are given less weight in the discussion that follows than are those for cobalt and open-heart surgery.

Except for the number at the top of each column, the numbers in the table represent the *differences in the probability of having the technology*

36. The distribution of the 2,772 hospitals for each of these factors is given in appendix A.

Table 5-2. The Probability That a Hospital Had Cobalt Therapy in 1975: Differences Associated with Selected Characteristics of the Hospital and Its Market[a]

	Probability	
Characteristic	Regression excluding third party payment	Regression including third party payment
Probability for hospitals with all the reference characteristics[b]	−0.003 (0.1)	−0.030 (0.7)
	Differences associated with size, control, and service	
Beds		
Under 100	Reference class	Reference class
100–199	+0.051 (2.7)**	+0.054 (2.9)**
200–299	+0.164 (7.6)**	+0.166 (7.7)**
300 and over	+0.469 (20.4)**	+0.475 (20.6)**
Control		
Private nonprofit	Reference class	Reference class
State and local government	−0.012 (0.6)	−0.012 (0.6)
Private, profit	−0.008 (0.4)	−0.013 (0.6)
Service		
General	Reference class	Reference class
Specialized	−0.063 (2.0)**	−0.061 (2.0)**
	Differences associated with teaching and research	
Medical school affiliation		
Yes	+0.114 (4.9)**	+0.115 (5.0)**
No	Reference class	Reference class
Residents per 100 beds		
0	Reference class	Reference class
1–9	+0.007 (0.4)	+0.012 (0.6)
10–19	+0.076 (2.4)**	+0.079 (2.5)**
20 and over	+0.169 (4.6)**	+0.171 (4.7)**
Research grants to hospitals, dollars per bed		
0	Reference class	Reference class
1–99	+0.032 (1.3)	+0.042 (1.7)*
100–999	+0.017 (0.7)	+0.025 (0.9)
1,000 and over	−0.011 (0.4)	+0.023 (0.7)
	Differences associated with patient care	
Doctors per 1,000 beds		
Under 175	+0.074 (3.3)**	+0.066 (2.8)**
175–249	Reference class	Reference class
250 and over	+0.042 (2.2)**	+0.019 (0.9)
Percent of doctors in general practice		
Under 20	−0.052 (2.1)**	−0.055 (2.2)**
20–29	Reference class	Reference class
30 and over	+0.012 (0.4)	−0.003 (0.1)

Table 5-2 (*continued*)

Characteristic	Probability	
	Regression excluding third party payment	*Regression including third party payment*
	Differences associated with patient care (continued)	
Percent of doctors in medical specialties		
Under 20	−0.018 (0.7)	−0.001 (0.0)
20–24	Reference class	Reference class
25 and over	−0.016 (0.8)	−0.005 (0.3)
Percent of doctors in surgical specialties		
Under 30	+0.027 (1.5)	+0.029 (1.5)
30–34	Reference class	Reference class
35 and over	+0.070 (3.1)**	+0.066 (2.8)**
Deaths from cancer per 1,000 beds		
Under 200	−0.030 (1.2)	−0.028 (1.0)
200–299	−0.014 (0.7)	−0.009 (0.4)
300–399	Reference class	Reference class
400 and over	+0.003 (0.1)	+0.004 (0.2)
Percent of population 65 years and older		
Under 10	Reference class	Reference class
10 and over	−0.008 (0.4)	−0.026 (1.1)
Percent of population white		
Under 85	−0.041 (2.1)**	−0.040 (1.8)*
85–94	Reference class	Reference class
95 and over	−0.054 (2.5)**	−0.056 (2.5)**
	Differences associated with market structure	
Percent of beds in four largest hospitals		
Under 50	Reference class	Reference class
50–79	−0.025 (1.1)	−0.028 (1.2)
80–100	+0.029 (1.1)	+0.025 (0.9)
Market with fewer than four hospitals	+0.025 (0.7)	+0.031 (0.8)
Percent growth in population, 1950–70		
Under 35	Reference class	Reference class
35–59	+0.039 (1.8)*	+0.041 (1.8)*
60 and over	+0.023 (0.9)	+0.019 (0.7)
	Differences associated with third party payment	
Percent of population with hospital insurance, 1963		
Under 65	...	−0.072 (1.8)*
65–74	...	−0.015 (0.4)
75–84	...	−0.002 (0.1)
85 and over	...	Reference class
Percent growth in hospital insurance, 1961–71		
Under 10	...	+0.020 (0.5)
10–19	...	Reference class
20–29	...	+0.060 (2.2)**
30 and over	...	+0.063 (2.0)**

Table 5-2 (*continued*)

Characteristic	Probability	
	Regression excluding third party payment	*Regression including third party payment*
	Differences associated with third party payment (*continued*)	
Percent of costs paid by Medicare		
Under 15	...	+0.015 (0.5)
15–19	...	−0.023 (1.1)
20–24	...	Reference class
25–29	...	+0.071 (2.9)**
30 and over	...	+0.017 (0.4)
	Differences associated with regulation	
Effective year, certificate-of-need law		
1965–69	−0.010 (0.3)	−0.014 (0.4)
1970–73	−0.040 (2.4)**	−0.036 (1.7)*
1974–75 or no law	Reference class	Reference class
Regional medical program dollars per hospital		
Under 100,000	Reference class	Reference class
100,000 and over	+0.030 (2.0)**	+0.015 (0.9)
Area comprehensive health planning dollars per hospital		
0	+0.001 (0.0)	+0.004 (0.2)
1–4,999	−0.026 (1.1)	−0.021 (0.9)
5,000–14,999	Reference class	Reference class
15,000 and over	−0.024 (1.2)	−0.003 (0.1)
Summary statistic		
Number of observations	2,772	2,772
R^2	0.351	0.357
Corrected R^2	0.342	0.346
F and degrees of freedom [numerator, denominator]	38.88 [38, 2733]	31.53 [48, 2723]

Sources: See chapter 2 for discussion of the basic data.
* The difference is statistically significant at the 90 percent level of confidence or better, but less than the 95 percent level.
** The difference is statistically significant at the 95 percent level of confidence or better.
a. The numbers in parentheses are *t*-statistics.
b. This is the constant term of the regression and shows the probability that applies to hospitals having all the reference characteristics. (See text for explanation of the notion of a reference class.)

(in 1975) associated with the various characteristics. For example, the number shown for hospitals with 100 through 199 beds in the first column of table 5-2, +0.051, means that the probability that hospitals of this size reported cobalt therapy in 1975 is greater by 0.051 than the probability for hospitals with fewer than 100 beds, the reference class. An alternative and equally valid interpretation is that the numbers show the differences in the *proportion* of the 2,772 hospitals that reported cobalt therapy and

Table 5-3. The Probability That a Hospital Had Open-Heart Surgery in 1975: Differences Associated with Selected Characteristics of the Hospital and Its Market[a]

	Probability	
Characteristic	*Regression excluding third party payment*	*Regression including third party payment*
Probability for hospitals with all the reference characteristics[b]	0.035 (1.0)	0.031 (0.8)
	Differences associated with size, control, and service	
Beds		
Under 100	Reference class	Reference class
100–199	+0.053 (3.2)**	+0.056 (3.4)**
200–299	+0.137 (7.2)**	+0.140 (7.3)**
300 and over	+0.270 (13.3)**	+0.274 (13.5)**
Control		
Private nonprofit	Reference class	Reference class
State and local government	−0.056 (3.3)**	−0.064 (3.8)**
Private, profit	−0.010 (0.6)	−0.028 (1.5)
Service		
General	Reference class	Reference class
Specialized	−0.001 (0.0)	−0.004 (0.1)
	Differences associated with teaching and research	
Medical school affiliation		
Yes	+0.225 (10.9)**	+0.224 (10.9)**
No	Reference class	Reference class
Residents per 100 beds		
0	Reference class	Reference class
1–9	+0.032 (1.8)*	+0.033 (1.8)*
10–19	+0.073 (2.6)**	+0.076 (2.7)**
20 and over	+0.386 (12.0)**	+0.387 (12.0)**
Research grants to hospitals, dollars per bed		
0	Reference class	Reference class
1–99	−0.025 (1.2)	−0.026 (1.2)
100–999	−0.001 (0.0)	+0.017 (0.7)
1,000 and over	−0.040 (1.5)	−0.028 (1.0)
	Differences associated with patient care	
Doctors per 1,000 beds		
Under 175	−0.060 (2.9)**	−0.052 (2.4)**
175–249	Reference class	Reference class
250 and over	+0.014 (0.8)	+0.005 (0.3)
Percent of doctors in general practice		
Under 20	+0.051 (2.4)**	+0.043 (2.0)**
20–29	Reference class	Reference class
30 and over	+0.027 (1.1)	+0.026 (1.0)
Percent of doctors in medical specialties		
Under 20	+0.016 (0.7)	+0.022 (0.9)
20–24	Reference class	Reference class
25 and over	−0.037 (2.0)**	−0.026 (1.3)

Table 5-3 (*continued*)

	Probability	
Characteristic	*Regression excluding third party payment*	*Regression including third party payment*

Differences associated with patient care (*continued*)

Percent of doctors in surgical specialties
Under 30	−0.016 (1.0)	−0.001 (0.7)
30–34	Reference class	Reference class
35 and over	+0.061 (3.1)**	+0.050 (2.3)**

Deaths from heart disease per 1,000 beds
Under 350	+0.075 (2.8)**	+0.066 (2.4)**
350–449	+0.000 (0.0)	+0.005 (0.2)
450–549	−0.015 (0.8)	−0.010 (0.5)
550–649	Reference class	Reference class
650 and over	−0.037 (1.8)*	−0.036 (1.6)

Percent of population 65 years and older
Under 10	Reference class	Reference class
10 and over	−0.020 (1.1)	−0.021 (1.0)

Percent of population white
Under 85	−0.064 (3.7)**	−0.086 (4.3)**
85–94	Reference class	Reference class
95 and over	−0.009 (0.5)	−0.003 (0.1)

Differences associated with market structure

Percent of beds in four largest hospitals
Under 50	Reference class	Reference class
50–79	−0.011 (0.6)	−0.013 (0.6)
80–100	−0.023 (1.0)	−0.026 (1.1)
Market with fewer than four hospitals	−0.073 (2.2)**	−0.072 (2.1)**

Percent growth in population, 1950–70
Under 35	Reference class	Reference class
35–59	+0.038 (1.9)*	+0.039 (1.9)*
60 and over	+0.085 (4.0)**	+0.067 (2.9)**

Differences associated with third party payment

Percent of population with hospital insurance, 1963
Under 65	...	−0.029 (0.8)
65–74	...	+0.007 (0.2)
75–84	...	−0.037 (1.3)
85 and over	...	Reference class

Percent growth in hospital insurance, 1961–71
Under 10	...	+0.036 (1.1)
10–19	...	Reference class
20–29	...	+0.012 (0.5)
30 and over	...	+0.061 (2.2)**

Table 5-3 (*continued*)

	Probability	
Characteristic	*Regression excluding third party payment*	*Regression including third party payment*
	Differences associated with third party payment (*continued*)	
Percent of costs paid by Medicare		
Under 15	...	+0.034 (1.2)
15–19	...	−0.018 (1.0)
20–24	...	Reference class
25–29	...	−0.017 (0.8)
30 and over	...	−0.004 (0.1)
	Differences associated with regulation	
Effective year, certificate-of-need law		
1965–69	−0.087 (3.3)**	−0.097 (3.0)**
1970–73	−0.027 (1.9)*	−0.013 (0.7)
1974–75 or no law	Reference class	Reference class
Regional medical program dollars per hospital		
Under 100,000	Reference class	Reference class
100,000 and over	−0.002 (0.1)	−0.016 (1.0)
Area comprehensive health planning dollars per hospital		
0	−0.019 (0.8)	−0.025 (1.0)
1–4,999	−0.046 (2.2)**	−0.047 (2.2)**
5,000–14,999	Reference class	Reference class
15,000 and over	−0.026 (1.5)	−0.021 (1.1)
Summary statistic		
Number of observations	2,772	2,772
R^2	0.386	0.392
Corrected R^2	0.378	0.381
F and degrees of freedom [numerator, denominator]	44.08 [39, 2732]	35.76 [49, 2722]

Sources: See chapter 2 for discussion of the basic data.
* The difference is statistically significant at the 90 percent level of confidence or better, but less than the 95 percent level.
** The difference is statistically significant at the 95 percent level of confidence or better.
a. The numbers in parentheses are *t*-statistics.
b. This is the constant term of the regression and shows the probability that applies to hospitals having all the reference characteristics. (See text for explanation of the notion of a reference class.)

that, for example, the proportion is 0.051 greater for hospitals with 100 through 199 beds, 0.164 greater for those with 200 through 299 beds, and so on. As before, these differences are added to or subtracted from the number at the top of each column, which is the probability (proportion) that applies to hospitals having all the characteristics of the reference classes. The resulting total is the probability (proportion) for hospitals with the characteristics selected.

Table 5-4. The Probability That a Hospital Had Renal Dialysis in 1975: Differences Associated with Selected Characteristics of the Hospital and Its Market[a]

	Probability	
Characteristic	Inpatient dialysis	Outpatient dialysis
Probability for hospitals with all the reference characteristics[b]	−0.092 (2.1)**	−0.042 (1.0)
Differences associated with size, control, and service		
Beds		
Under 100	Reference class	Reference class
100–199	+0.074 (4.0)**	+0.043 (2.5)**
200–299	+0.183 (8.4)**	+0.113 (5.6)**
300 and over	+0.333 (14.3)**	+0.238 (11.0)**
Control		
Private nonprofit	Reference class	Reference class
State and local government	−0.005 (0.3)	+0.010 (0.6)
Private, profit	−0.015 (0.7)	−0.007 (0.3)
Service		
General	Reference class	Reference class
Specialized	−0.122 (3.9)**	−0.091 (3.1)**
Differences associated with teaching and research		
Medical school affiliation		
Yes	+0.176 (7.5)**	+0.163 (7.5)**
No	Reference class	Reference class
Residents per 100 beds		
0	Reference class	Reference class
1–9	+0.045 (2.2)**	+0.016 (0.8)
10–19	+0.142 (4.4)**	+0.118 (4.0)**
20 and over	+0.351 (9.5)**	+0.399 (11.7)**
Research grants to hospitals, dollars per bed		
0	Reference class	Reference class
1–99	−0.012 (0.5)	+0.004 (0.2)
100–999	−0.003 (0.1)	+0.020 (0.8)
1,000 and over	+0.005 (0.2)	+0.032 (1.1)
Differences associated with patient care		
Doctors per 1,000 beds		
Under 175	−0.031 (1.2)	+0.008 (0.4)
175–249	Reference class	Reference class
250 and over	+0.020 (0.9)	−0.014 (0.7)
Percent of doctors in general practice		
Under 20	+0.063 (2.5)**	+0.038 (1.7)*
20–29	Reference class	Reference class
30 and over	−0.027 (0.9)	−0.015 (0.6)

Table 5-4 (*continued*)

Characteristic	Probability	
	Inpatient dialysis	*Outpatient dialysis*
	Differences associated with patient care (*continued*)	
Percent of doctors in medical specialties		
Under 20	+0.087 (3.0)**	+0.043 (1.6)
20–24	Reference class	Reference class
25 and over	−0.001 (0.1)	−0.018 (0.9)
Percent of doctors in surgical specialties		
Under 30	+0.043 (2.2)**	+0.009 (0.5)
30–34	Reference class	Reference class
35 and over	+0.013 (0.5)	+0.001 (0.0)
Population per bed		
Under 200	−0.025 (1.0)	−0.031 (1.4)
200–249	Reference class	Reference class
250–299	−0.042 (2.0)**	−0.029 (1.5)
300 and over	−0.053 (1.8)*	+0.011 (0.4)
Percent of population 65 years and older		
Under 10	Reference class	Reference class
10 and over	+0.015 (0.6)	−0.000 (0.0)
Percent of population white		
Under 85	−0.011 (0.5)	−0.016 (0.8)
85–94	Reference class	Reference class
95 and over	+0.026 (1.1)	+0.015 (0.7)
	Differences associated with market structure	
Percent of beds in four largest hospitals		
Under 50	Reference class	Reference class
50–79	−0.008 (0.4)	+0.006 (0.3)
80–100	+0.018 (0.7)	+0.040 (1.6)
Market with fewer than four hospitals	+0.018 (0.5)	+0.075 (2.1)**
Percent growth in population, 1950–70		
Under 35	Reference class	Reference class
35–59	+0.041 (1.8)*	+0.026 (1.2)
60 and over	+0.094 (3.4)**	+0.053 (2.1)**
	Differences associated with third party payment	
Percent of population with hospital insurance, 1963		
Under 65	+0.033 (0.8)	+0.011 (0.3)
65–74	+0.060 (1.8)*	+0.018 (0.6)
75–84	−0.005 (0.2)	−0.022 (0.8)
85 and over	Reference class	Reference class
Percent growth in hospital insurance, 1961–71		
Under 10	+0.092 (2.5)**	+0.079 (2.3)**
10–19	Reference class	Reference class
20–29	+0.029 (1.0)	+0.061 (2.3)**
30 and over	+0.049 (1.5)	+0.037 (1.2)

Table 5-4 (*continued*)

Characteristic	Probability	
	Inpatient dialysis	*Outpatient dialysis*
	Differences associated with third party payment (*continued*)	
Percent of costs paid by Medicare		
Under 15	−0.046 (1.4)	−0.075 (2.5)**
15–19	−0.023 (1.1)	−0.035 (1.8)*
20–24	Reference class	Reference class
25–29	−0.007 (0.3)	−0.003 (0.1)
30 and over	−0.062 (1.6)	−0.054 (1.5)
	Differences associated with regulation	
Effective year, certificate-of-need law		
1965–69	−0.032 (0.9)	−0.035 (1.0)
1970–73	−0.020 (0.9)	−0.012 (0.6)
1974–75 or no law	Reference class	Reference class
Regional medical program dollars per hospital		
Under 100,000	Reference class	Reference class
100,000 and over	−0.004 (0.2)	+0.005 (0.3)
Area comprehensive health planning dollars per hospital		
0	−0.014 (0.5)	−0.020 (0.8)
1–4,999	−0.006 (0.3)	−0.017 (0.8)
5,000–14,999	Reference class	Reference class
15,000 and over	−0.003 (0.1)	−0.020 (1.0)
Summary statistic		
Number of observations	2,772	2,772
R^2	0.335	0.301
Corrected R^2	0.324	0.289
F and degrees of freedom [numerator, denominator]	28.59 [48, 2723]	24.41 [48, 2723]

Sources: See chapter 2 for discussion of the basic data.

* The difference is statistically significant at the 90 percent level of confidence or better, but less than the 95 percent level.

** The difference is statistically significant at the 95 percent level of confidence or better.

a. The numbers in parentheses are *t*-statistics.

b. This is the constant term of the regression and shows the probability that applies to hospitals having all the reference characteristics. (See text for explanation of the notion of a reference class.)

By definition, probabilities and proportions must lie between zero and one.[37] But the reader will note that the probabilities shown at the top of tables 5-2 and 5-4—which, again, are the probabilities that apply to hospitals having all the reference characteristics—are negative, although they

37. For a probability, zero means that the event has no chance of occurring and one means that it is certain to occur. For a proportion, the interpretations are a little different: zero means that none of the hospitals with the specified characteristics had the technology, one that all of them did.

are statistically insignificant in every case except inpatient dialysis.[38] As a practical matter, these values should be interpreted as probabilities of zero, as should any negative estimates that might result from adding together the differences for particular combinations of characteristics.

For all three technologies the number of beds in the hospital—which is a first approximation to the scale of operation of all its activities—is a very important determinant of whether it adopted the technology by 1975. The larger the hospital, the more likely it is to have the technology, and each additional 100 beds makes a substantial difference to the probability. For hospitals with fewer than 300 beds, the differences are rather similar across technologies; but for those with 300 beds or more, sheer scale has been much more important to the adoption of cobalt therapy than the others. The probability that a hospital of this size—but with the characteristics of the reference classes in all other respects—has cobalt therapy is about 0.45 (0.469 less 0.003 in column 1 of table 5-2, 0.475 less 0.030 in column 2), compared to probabilities of about 0.20 through 0.25 for open-heart surgery and both forms of renal dialysis.

For the most part, the type of organization that controls the hospital has no effect; the only exception is that state and local government hospitals are substantially less likely to have an open-heart surgery unit. The type of service provided by the hospital is more important. Specialized hospitals are much less likely to have cobalt therapy or renal dialysis in either form than general service hospitals, but there is no difference between the two types of hospital in the probability of having open-heart surgery. This is consistent, for one, with the types of diseases treated by children's hospitals, a major type of specialty hospital—children rarely develop cancer or kidney failure but are more frequently born with heart defects, which can be corrected by surgery.

Teaching programs have had an extremely important influence on the adoption of all three technologies, particularly open-heart surgery: affiliation with a medical school raises the probability that a hospital has this technology by 0.22, and the probability grows as the number of residents per 100 beds increases, with twenty or more residents per 100 beds asso-

---

38. This outcome is always possible when, as here, ordinary least squares is used to estimate an equation in which the dependent variable is binary, that is, takes either the value one (has the technology) or zero (does not have the technology). The problem could have been avoided by using one of several special estimating techniques, but each of these has its own problems and limitations. On the whole, the costs seemed greater than the benefits, and ordinary least squares was used instead. The arguments are reviewed in appendix B.

ciated with an increase of nearly 0.40 over the reference class (no residents). In essence, a large hospital affiliated with a medical school and committed to an extensive program of residency training is virtually certain to have an open-heart surgery unit (taking the numbers from column 1 of table 5-3, $0.035 + 0.270 + 0.225 + 0.386 = 0.916$). The effects of these factors are nearly as impressive for renal dialysis but much less so for cobalt therapy, where, as noted, size alone seems to have been more important in determining adoption. Greater or lesser commitment to research as measured by grant dollars per bed appears to have added nothing to the more general influence of medical school affiliation on the adoption of these technologies.

The factors under the patient care heading include both the characteristics of doctors and the incidence of disease in the population. And from the hospital's point of view, the two may be nearly indistinguishable: patients who come to the hospital are, for the most part, those the affiliated doctors recommend for admission, and the hospital may not have much independent information about its potential patients nor any way to get to them except through the doctors.

The adoption of both cobalt therapy and open-heart surgery has been influenced by the number and specialty distribution of the doctors in the hospital's market area but not always in the same way. Open-heart surgery has been adopted more often where there are more doctors, as indicated by the estimates showing that it is less likely in areas with fewer than 175 doctors per 1,000 hospital beds; there is no difference between hospitals in areas with 175 through 249 doctors and areas with 250 or more doctors. Cobalt therapy, on the other hand, is more common in the areas with the fewest doctors than in the other areas.

Quite logically, since radiation often follows surgery for cancer and open-heart surgery is a surgical procedure, both technologies have been adopted more often by hospitals in areas with a relative abundance of surgeons. When 35 percent or more of the doctors in the area are in the surgical specialties, the probability of having the technology, or alternatively the proportion of hospitals reporting it, is higher by 0.07 for cobalt therapy and by 0.05 to 0.06 for open-heart surgery.

For open-heart surgery, the remaining specialties are a passive reflection of the positive correlation with surgeons. The probability is less where there are relatively more doctors in general practice or in the medical specialties. But cobalt therapy is actually found more frequently, rather than less, where there are more physicians in general practice; this is shown by the reduced probability for hospitals in areas where fewer than 20 percent of the doctors are in general practice. One possible, but quite tentative, explanation is that, because cobalt therapy is an older technology, it has been completely accepted by doctors and, in fact, has reached the point where it is no longer considered quite the thing by those who are more specialized and who work on the frontiers of radiation therapy and cancer treatment. This is consistent with the fact that teaching hospitals in particular look upon linear accelerators as newer and better than cobalt and with recent literature that emphasizes the advantages of high-energy accelerators over cobalt.[39]

None of the three technologies shows any marked tendency to have been adopted more frequently where the incidence of the related diseases —approximated by cancer deaths in the case of cobalt therapy, heart disease deaths in the case of open-heart surgery, and population in the case of renal dialysis—is higher. The relationship between the adoption of cobalt therapy and deaths from cancer is in the right direction but is so slight that it is not statistically significant at any point. The relationship between open-heart surgery and deaths from heart disease is significant but not in the expected direction: open-heart surgery units have been adopted more frequently where there are fewer deaths from heart disease. It might be tempting to conclude that the relationship is causal—that open-heart surgery reduces deaths from heart disease—but the years covered by the data, 1968 through 1971, rule out this interpretation for this period. Open-heart surgery, and particularly the bypass procedure, was just getting started in those years and had not been around long enough or done frequently enough to have had any measurable effect on mortality statistics for the entire population. Instead, the results must be interpreted as meaning that hospitals did not respond to the local incidence of heart disease in deciding to adopt an open-heart surgery unit and that the factors they did respond to produced a pattern in which units are more common in areas where mortality is already lower.

The proportion of people sixty-five years old or older has had no influence on the adoption of any of the technologies. The effect of the racial composition of the population varies with the technology—cobalt therapy

39. The results in table 5-4 indicate that inpatient dialysis is adopted more often where there are fewer doctors in all three specialty groups—general practice, medical, and surgical. When these were replaced by the residual "other specialties" group, to test whether they pointed to a relationship with that group, the results were statistically insignificant.

is less common both where the proportion of whites is especially low and where it is especially high, open-heart surgery is less common where it is especially low, and renal dialysis is unaffected. The results for cobalt therapy hint that this characteristic may represent some factor other than, or in addition to, race.

The degree of competition in the hospital's market, measured by the four-firm concentration ratio, is important for open-heart surgery but not for cobalt therapy. Open-heart surgery units have been adopted more frequently in competitive markets than in highly concentrated ones: the probability of having this technology declines steadily as the market grows more concentrated. This result is unique in the study. The concentration ratio showed no relationship with the technologies considered in chapters 3 and 4.[40]

For all three technologies, hospitals in markets where the population has grown most quickly are more likely to have the technology. For open-heart surgery, for example, the probability is about 0.04 higher for a hospital in a market whose population grew between 35 and 60 percent in the years from 1950 to 1970 than for a hospital in a market where the growth was less than 35 percent (table 5-3). And where the growth was 60 percent or more, the probability increases by about 0.07 or 0.08.

In spite of their inadequacies, all of the measures of third party payment behave as expected in the case of cobalt therapy. Hospitals in areas that had lower levels of insurance coverage in 1963 adopted cobalt therapy less readily, and the differences are larger the lower the level of coverage —with that for the lowest level, less than 65 percent, significant at the 90 percent level. Further, where insurance growth was greater, hospitals have been more likely to adopt cobalt therapy; the differences for the two highest growth classes (20 through 29 percent and 30 percent or more) are both substantial and significant. The Medicare data work in the same direction. Hospitals in areas where Medicare paid 25 through 29 percent of all hospital costs are more likely to have adopted cobalt therapy than those in areas where Medicare paid less than 25 percent. The highest class, 30 percent or more, does not fit the pattern but, as chapter 2 points out, the percentages in this range are probably overstated in many cases, since

40. The results in table 5-4 suggest that hospitals in more concentrated markets are *more* likely to have outpatient dialysis. If this is not simply an artifact, it may reflect a situation in which at least one hospital in a market generally takes responsibility for establishing a unit because it is particularly important for dialysis patients that these facilities be nearby.

they are most affected by payments to extended-care facilities. Finally, the plausibility of the results is heightened by the fact that when third party payment was included, two rather odd results that appeared when it was left out, disappeared—a U-shaped relationship with number of doctors per 1,000 beds and a positive difference for well-funded regional medical programs.

The pattern is not true of open-heart surgery or renal dialysis. For open-heart surgery, the probability of having the technology is significantly higher in areas with the highest growth in insurance coverage, but neither the level of insurance in 1963 nor the share of costs paid by Medicare is important. In the case of dialysis there is no consistent pattern and significant differences are as often in the wrong direction as the right one.

The regional medical program has had no effect on the adoption of these technologies—not even renal dialysis, the one promoted most energetically by the program. Similarly, the area comprehensive health planning agencies have had no effect on the adoption of cobalt therapy or renal dialysis, but there is a suggestion that some of these agencies may have helped to encourage the adoption of open-heart surgery. The probability of having a unit is lower for hospitals in areas where the agencies had less than $5,000 per hospital to spend, compared to the reference class ($5,000 through $14,999). But the pattern is muddied considerably by the fact that the difference for those with the most money is also negative and, while not significant at the conventional levels, both large enough and significant enough to mean that the difference between the areas with the least funds and those with the most is insignificant. In the absence of any support in the rest of the analysis for the influence of these agencies, the results for open-heart surgery should not be taken too seriously.

The results for certificate-of-need laws are quite interesting. It is observed in chapter 2 that if these reviews have had an effect, that effect may well have varied with the technology and the state, since it would have depended on what the reviewers perceived as good and bad technologies. It would have depended as well on the number of applications they got for a particular technology—they do not have the power to order the removal of facilities.

Certificate-of-need laws have had no effect on the adoption of renal dialysis, consistent with the facts that it was and is widely perceived as a technology with clear and worthwhile benefits and that it was still in its heyday in the early 1970s. The results for cobalt therapy suggest that in New York, which accounts for most of the hospitals in the 1965–69 class, the review board either has not discouraged the adoption of cobalt therapy or, perhaps more likely, has not had the opportunity to do so. Many New York hospitals are large teaching hospitals, in the vanguard of technical change, and they may well have been moving on to linear accelerators by the time the law went into effect in 1965. But in states with more recent laws, the reviews have succeeded in discouraging the adoption of cobalt therapy by a modest (-0.04) but statistically significant amount.

Certificate-of-need laws appear to have had a more general depressing effect on open-heart surgery. The early laws reduced the probability that a hospital had adopted open-heart surgery by 1975 quite substantially, by about -0.09. The later laws also appear to have had some effect, again rather modest, in keeping with the shorter length of time available to them to review applications for this technology; but the difference is not statistically significant when third party payment is included.

This chapter completes the statistical analysis. Again, patterns have appeared that appeared in chapters 3 and 4. But before these common patterns are reviewed in the final chapter, chapter 7, government policies toward hospital technologies in the United States and three other countries are considered in chapter 6.

Technical Note

The regressions for renal dialysis are not as successful as those for cobalt therapy and open-heart surgery. Aside from scale, service, and teaching, the differences tend either to be insignificant or to form patterns that are not very informative (for example, the results for the specialties of physicians). There are several possible reasons for this outcome:

1. In the years just before 1975 renal dialysis was being adopted faster than cobalt therapy (which had reached a plateau) and open-heart surgery (which was spreading slowly). The analysis is aimed at explaining an equilibrium or final level of adoption and it may be that, for renal dialysis, the 1975 level is not a good approximation to this level.

2. The fact that renal dialysis was still spreading in the early 1970s further suggests that some of the influences on it may have been more recent than the data used in the analysis.

3. Outpatient dialysis is better measured by the number of dialysis stations in a unit than by simply whether the hospital had a unit. The analysis of intensive care beds (chapter 3) shows how useful this kind of measure

can be, and the crudeness of the dialysis measure may be another reason for the rather disappointing results.

4. A sizable minority of outpatient dialysis facilities are neither in, nor under the management of, hospitals. It may be that trying to explain adoption by hospitals without reference to these other facilities is too great an omission and distorts the results.

chapter six **Guiding Diffusion: Public Policies in the United States and Other Countries**

The United States is not alone in facing the dilemmas posed by medical technologies. The industrialized nations in general share the philosophy that no one should have to forgo care for lack of money. They have put this ideal into practice through a variety of institutions— private insurance, government financing, government-operated health services, and combinations and permutations of these. Their common ideal has brought them common problems. As the case studies of individual technologies show, there are a great many things worth doing in medical care if the only test is that they confer *some* benefit on the patient, however small or costly. It is very expensive to do all of them.

Faced with rapidly rising expenditures for medical care, governments have intervened increasingly in the process of marshaling resources for use in medical care. This chapter examines the form intervention has taken in four countries—the United States, Sweden, Great Britain, and France. In keeping with the subject of the study, it examines laws and policies that have important implications for the distribution of medical technologies. Not all of these laws and policies are directed explicitly at medical technologies, although some of them are, but in every case they are directed at the use of resources—usually capital resources—in such a way that technologies are inevitably one of their major targets. The purposes of these descriptions of policy are to demonstrate the prevalence of the problem, by demonstrating the prevalence of attempts to deal with it, and to indicate how far these countries have developed their thinking about it.

The latter point is clearest when the various forms of intervention are viewed as responses to a hierarchy of policy concerns. Each step of the hierarchy represents a growing commitment to cost containment over other goals—starting at the lowest step with no concern about cost at all— and together they provide a useful framework for comparing different

132

countries and for judging the extent to which their policies deal with the questions central to cost control.

Starting at the first, and least controversial, step of the hierarchy, governments may try to promote the adoption of new technologies. In the belief that a particular technology is a good thing, they may try to shorten the natural lags that impede its diffusion. For example, they might help pay for the equipment. They might publish information about its use or about the various models on the market to make it easier for patients, doctors, and hospital administrators to become familiar with it, and, as a consequence, to become comfortable about using it. They might train people to use the technology.

Moving up the hierarchy to step number two, governments may concern themselves with whether new technologies are being used efficiently, in what economists like to call the technical or engineering sense of that word.[1] Without making judgments about the volume of use, they may ask whether that volume is being produced at the lowest possible cost. Are existing facilities used to capacity? Are they large enough to take full advantage of any economies of scale? Are they run by people with enough training, but not too much? Is there "unnecessary" duplication? Considerations of geographic equity and of patient travel times may be brought into the deliberations, and will help determine how much duplication is "necessary" and how much underuse is, in the last analysis, perhaps desirable. Intervention on behalf of greater efficiency is based, of course, on the premise that the unregulated situation is not acceptably efficient and that intervention can improve matters.

These first two steps take as given that the technology is a good thing, that it is beneficial for patients in some fashion and therefore worth having. Implicitly, judgments about benefits are left to the medical profession, individually and collectively, and to patients. Whatever information they absorb is assumed to be correct.

But, in fact, the value of many medical practices has not been proven.[2]

1. In this chapter, the words "efficiency" and "efficiently" are used in this sense.
2. A. L. Cochrane, *Effectiveness and Efficiency: Random Reflections on Health Services* (London: Nuffield Provincial Hospitals Trust, 1972); Howard H. Hiatt, "Protecting the Medical Commons: Who Is Responsible?" *New England Journal of Medicine*, vol. 293 (July 31, 1975), pp. 235–41; Alan K. Pierce and Herbert A. Saltzman, "Conference on the Scientific Basis of Respiratory Therapy," in *Proceedings of the Conference on the Scientific Basis of Respiratory Therapy*, pt. 2 of *American Review of Respiratory Disease*, vol. 110 (December 1974), pp. 1–15; Paul D. Stolley, "Assuring the Safety and Efficacy of Therapies," *International Journal of Health Services*, vol. 4 (Winter 1974), pp. 131–45.

The enthusiasms of one era are often discredited in the next. Thus the third step of the hierarchy gets the government into the business of questioning, even testing, the benefits of medical technologies. The simplest way to approach this problem is to make the previously implicit process explicit, and to ask, Does the medical profession, or its most prestigious representatives in the appropriate field, think that the technology is beneficial, and for whom? This approach can take the form of expert conferences that try to arrive at guidelines for the individual physician or of review committees that examine the care given individual patients and recommend, or even enforce, changes.

This still assumes, of course, that whatever steps the profession has taken to learn about the benefits of various technologies are sufficient to support the judgments that are made. The government may decide to question this assumption too, and ask, Has the technology been proven beneficial by persuasive scientific evidence, particularly in the form of randomized controlled trials? In a randomized controlled trial patients are randomly assigned to a group that receives the new treatment or to a group that receives alternative treatments or a placebo. Objective criteria for success or failure are established at the outset and the trial is designed, if possible, to keep the patients and doctors from knowing which groups are receiving the new treatment, which the alternatives. The point of this last safeguard is to avoid the possibility that the outcome will be influenced by doctors' and patients' beliefs about which alternative is best.

When the government establishes by either expert opinion or controlled trial that a technology is *not* beneficial, it may try to devise means to prevent its use. This is perhaps easiest to do if the technology requires a piece of capital equipment whose purchase can be forbidden. A variation on this approach is to ask which of several more or less equally beneficial alternatives is cheapest and to try to encourage the use of that alternative and the abandonment of the others.

Step number four in the hierarchy brings the government to the crux of the cost problem and into a storm of controversy. At this step, the government explicitly accepts the possibility that it may not be unquestionably desirable to provide every kind of care that has some benefit, however small or costly. The question shifts from, Is it beneficial? to, Is it beneficial *enough?* Are the benefits of the technology enough to justify the costs? The government need not adopt the position that the cutoff point should be the same as that which would be observed in an ordinary market in which the patient paid the full cost of care out of his own pocket.

But in moving into this area, it leaves behind the philosophy that everything that is needed, in the sense that it can reasonably be expected to confer some benefit on the patient, will be provided, and accepts the philosophy that some things are so costly in comparison to their benefits that a society faced with limited resources may decide that those resources could be put to better use elsewhere.

From a cursory glance at a number of countries it appears that most have been inclined to stay close to the lower end of the hierarchy, taking the level of services as given and concerning themselves primarily with keeping the costs of those services down. This may reflect the fact that the problems—the rapid growth of costs in general, and the arrival of a number of expensive new technologies in particular—are relatively recent, at least in their serious form. Much of the legislation and policy discussed here is, therefore, also relatively recent: the United States passed its national health planning law in 1974, the French their hospital reform act in 1970.

Rather by accident than design, the four countries discussed in this chapter cover the entire range of possibilities, including the seldom-seen top of the hierarchy. The information about them comes from published articles and books and from less accessible literature supplied by people in the countries concerned. The choice was based in large part on the availability and language of this literature rather than because of the, happily excellent, ability of these particular four to illustrate the steps of the hierarchy.

For the most part, the following sections describe what is on paper—laws, procedures, reporting requirements, policy statements. What exists in reality can look considerably different. (Of course, where the legislation or policy is recent, there has hardly been time for the ideal to influence practice at all.) It would involve a great deal of work, going well beyond the scope of a single chapter, to produce a good study of the reality in each case. But wherever possible, bits and pieces of reality have been brought in so that the reader can, if not judge, at least suspect the divergences and come to a more realistic appraisal of the potential of the ideal.

As background for the discussions of policy, it is useful to compare the resources committed to medical care in the four countries—to suggest the extent to which each has encouraged or restrained the flow of resources into this sector of its economy. The measure usually employed is the percent of gross national product a country spends on medical care. This is an approximate measure and estimates vary from source to source. Prob-

Table 6-1. Estimates of Expenditures for Health Services as a Percent of Gross National Product, Selected Countries, 1968, 1969, and 1975

Country	1975	1969	1968
United States	8.4	6.8	7.5
Sweden	9.2	6.7	8.1
United Kingdom[a]	5.4	4.8	5.2
France	8.1	5.7	n.a.

Sources: The 1975 numbers are unofficial estimates by the Social Security Administration, published in Victor Cohn and Peter Milius, "They Make Good by Making Well," *Washington Post*, January 7, 1979. The 1969 estimates are from Joseph G. Simanis, "Medical Care Expenditures in Seven Countries," *Social Security Bulletin*, vol. 36 (March 1973), table 1. The 1968 estimates are from Odin W. Anderson, *Health Care: Can There Be Equity? The United States, Sweden, and England* (Wiley, 1972), table A-6. Anderson estimates that if expenditures made outside the National Health Service were included, the figure for the United Kingdom would be increased by half a percentage point.
n.a. Not available.
a. The United Kingdom includes Great Britain (England, Wales, and Scotland) and Northern Ireland.

ably the major reason for the differences is the simplest: it is difficult to find all the necessary statistics for each country and to maintain a consistent definition of medical care in the face of the variations in the way different countries provide care.

Table 6-1 shows estimates for 1968, 1969, and 1975. The numbers for 1968 and 1969 are from different authors, using different sources and methods, and indicate the imprecision of the estimates. But the rank order among countries would elicit considerable agreement. Great Britain is generally believed to commit a lower percentage of its gross national product to medical care than most industrialized countries, including the other three in the table. Sweden and the United States are believed to have among the highest percentages, with Sweden edging ahead in recent years. Two other leaders, not discussed in this chapter, are West Germany and the Netherlands, which devoted 9.3 percent and 8.7 percent of their national resources to medical care in 1975.

The United States

The Heart Disease, Cancer, and Stroke Amendments of 1965, which established the regional medical program, were the first federal legislation aimed at influencing the distribution of medical technology and are, to date, the only legislation with that as its explicit purpose. At one time or another there were fifty-nine separate programs covering large areas within states or even crossing the boundaries of several states. Their job was to promote the use of new techniques for caring for patients with heart disease, cancer, and stroke, in order to shorten the time it takes for research to translate into practice, and to promote, as well, cooperative arrangements among institutions in the region to achieve this end.[3]

Training programs—for example, programs to educate nurses and physicians about coronary care and the use of coronary care units—were one of their major activities.[4] When kidney disease was added to the list in 1970, the development of dialysis centers and of cooperative regional networks for kidney donation and transplantation became important. But the program was overtaken by events. Promoting technologies began to seem like the wrong tack in a world of rapidly rising medical care costs, and the 1970 and 1972 amendments to the program turned it sharply away from its original purposes toward a much vaguer and more diffuse set: providing primary care in underserved areas, improving the quality of care and the productivity of medical manpower, and so on. The program that died in 1975 bore little resemblance to the one born in 1965.

The Comprehensive Health Planning and Public Health Services Amendments of 1966 established the idea of planning the use of all health resources, not just certain technologies, for the population of an area or a region. The law authorized the selection of state agencies and area agencies within states to undertake this planning. The agencies were provided with some federal money, no power, and remarkably little direction as to what they were to do or how they were to do it. Their general charge, "to promote the development of a healthful environment and a health care system in which quality health services would be available, accessible and affordable for all persons"[5] left nothing out. Each agency was to inventory the health resources in its area and draw up a plan for their future development. What those plans were to accomplish was left to local discretion at first. But in 1973 the federal government did suggest that certain objectives should be given greater weight; by that time, efficiency aimed at controlling costs seemed most important.[6]

From the perspective of medical technology, the most interesting development to grow out of the experience with comprehensive health planning—or, perhaps more accurately, to be intertwined with it—was the growth of state certificate-of-need laws. These laws, which gave planning

3. See *National Health Planning and Development and Health Facilities Assistance Act of 1974*, S. Rept. 93-1285, 93 Cong 2 sess. (Government Printing Office, 1974), pp. 13–18.

4. Nancy Kay, "The Regional Medical Programs: Contributions to Technological Diffusion" (unpublished paper available from author).

5. *National Health Planning*, S. Rept. 93-1285, p. 9.

6. Ibid., p. 12.

agencies their first and often only power, require that proposed investments in health facilities be reviewed by a state agency and approved only if the agency decides there is a need for the investment; review by the area planning agency is usually a required part of the process. New York passed the first certificate-of-need law in 1964. By the end of 1970 five states had enacted laws, and, in part with the help of the planning agencies, the number of state laws began to grow rapidly (see chapter 2, table 2-16). The details of the different state laws vary, but most cover all types of health facilities except doctors' offices and require approval of all new facilities, services, and equipment. Some states exempt projects that cost less than a specified amount, although this exemption often does not apply to projects that increase the bed capacity of an institution.

As it turned out, then, the comprehensive health planning program served as a bridge over a decade during which the goal of promoting technologies gave way to the goal of improving efficiency. The program did not last under its own name, but its principles survived intact in the National Health Planning and Resources Development Act of 1974, which designates state health planning agencies and approximately 200 health systems agencies. The health systems agencies closely resemble the old area agencies, and in fact in many cases one simply evolved into the other. The areas under their jurisdiction are supposed to be medical-care catchment areas, preferably with populations of more than 500,000 and less than 3 million, and self-sufficient enough that agencies can draw up plans focused on their areas. Each area agency is required to prepare a plan for the development of health resources and review it at least yearly. These area plans form the basis for the state plan prepared by the state agency.

The 1974 law requires each state to pass certificate-of-need legislation, with certain minimum features prescribed by the Department of Health, Education, and Welfare, and to do reviews. The agencies are no longer entirely free to choose their own objectives and guidelines. Although the objectives stated in the law itself are still a laundry list of conflicting possibilities, the Department of Health, Education, and Welfare, in conjunction with the National Council on Health Planning and Development established by the law, is required to promulgate more specific national guidelines, including "standards respecting the appropriate supply, distribution, and organization of health resources"[7] and to formulate them, as much as possible, in quantitative terms.

7. National Health Planning and Resources Development Act of 1974, sec. 1501(b)(1).

The first guidelines were published in March 1978, after long delays and a protracted and lively process of review and comment.[8] They set the standard for nonfederal short-term hospital beds (the law does not apply to federal facilities) at a maximum of four per 1,000 persons in the agency's area, with an occupancy rate of at least 80 percent. The remaining guidelines (for obstetrical inpatient services, neonatal special care units, pediatric inpatient services, open-heart surgery units, cardiac catheterization units, radiation therapy, computed tomography scanners, and renal dialysis) emphasize occupancy rates and minimum numbers of cases rather than ratios of facilities to population.[9] For example, the standard for open-heart surgery states that, within three years of the introduction of the unit, an institution for adults should perform 200 procedures a year and an institution for children, 75. This approach is considerably different from the one used in France (described later in this chapter) and has already been criticized for its potential for creating incentives for "overuse." Each standard sets out grounds for deviations—travel distances in sparsely populated rural areas, for example, or an unusually high proportion of elderly people in the area.

Meanwhile, the states' unguided application of their certificate-of-need laws—and related reviews carried out under the Social Security Amendments of 1972[10]—has formed in its collectivity the most important part of U.S. policy toward the distribution of medical technologies. The states have reviewed numerous applications for new services and equipment, but, not surprisingly, no general national policy has emerged from their separate experiences. There are many reasons for this, not the least of which are differences in objectives. Some state agencies viewed cost control as their major objective and tried to promote it through guidelines aimed at efficiency—the second step of the hierarchy described in the introduction—while other agencies considered their primary goal to be that of helping to bring more and better resources into the area.[11]

There have been two influences on this review process that deserve mention. One is Roemer's "law," a well-known statement in medical eco-

8. *Federal Register,* vol. 43 (March 28, 1978), pt. 4, pp. 13040–50.

9. The standard for renal dialysis simply states that providers should meet Medicare coverage requirements; these requirements, published elsewhere, prescribe minimum numbers of dialysis stations for a unit and minimum rates of use.

10. Sec. 1122 of the Social Security Act, added by the Social Security Amendments of 1972, sec. 221(a).

11. Lewin and Associates, *Evaluation of the Efficiency and Effectiveness of the Section 1122 Review Process,* pt. 1, prepared for the Health Resources Administration, Department of Health, Education, and Welfare (HRA, September 1975).

nomics, which says that in the presence of extensive third party coverage of medical care costs there is no practical limit to the number of hospital beds which, if available, can be filled with patients. The policy implications that have been drawn from Roemer's law are clear, simple, and easy to use. The most important one is that there are probably already enough hospital beds in any given area—perhaps too many—and regulators should hold the line against additions. This has focused regulators' attention on controlling hospital beds as the way to control capital investment, and through investment, annual operating costs in hospitals.[12]

The disadvantage of Roemer's law is that it implicitly assumes that other capital investment bears a fixed ratio to beds, so that to control beds is to control all that is important in hospital capacity and capital investment. This is clearly not the case. At best, then, Roemer's law is only a partial guide for the regulation of hospital investment and, by extension, for the control of operating expenses, since the connection between capital and operating expenses also undoubtedly has a great deal of play in it.

The pitfalls are illustrated by the experience of the Massachusetts certificate-of-need agency.[13] During its first nineteen months of existence, the agency reduced the overall number of beds in applicant hospitals by twenty-five, while permitting the number of intensive care beds to increase by eleven. The operating costs associated with intensive care beds are at least three times the costs of ward beds (see chapter 3). With its second move, the agency more than made up for any cost savings that might have resulted from its first.

The second influence on the review of technologies is the fact that, precisely because there is no Roemer's law for technologies, decisions about them are very hard to make. A great deal of information is needed and is not available—and without information about indications for use, benefits, existing facilities and their use, and other factors, any negative decision the review agency makes is an easy target for its opponents. Most agencies are much too small to collect the available information, let alone to generate the missing information. And since information does not produce agreement on objectives, the agency is still likely to find itself under

12. Herbert E. Klarman, "National Policies and Local Planning for Health Services," *Milbank Memorial Fund Quarterly: Health and Society,* vol. 54 (Winter 1976), p. 18.

13. William J. Bicknell and Diana Chapman Walsh, "Certification-of-need: The Massachusetts Experience," *New England Journal of Medicine,* vol. 292 (May 15, 1975), p. 1056.

fire. Altogether, between the focus on beds suggested by Roemer's law and the difficulty of developing grounds for denying requests for technologies, it is not surprising that these requests have generally been approved without the close review given to applications for new beds.[14]

The evidence of this study is that, even in the face of such difficulties, certificate-of-need reviews have had an effect on some technologies in some states where the perceptions and objectives of reviewers joined together with opportunity to permit it. States with laws that went into effect between 1965 and 1969 (most notably New York) reduced the proportion of hospital beds committed to intensive care below what it would have been otherwise (see chapter 3). States with laws that became effective between 1970 and 1973 discouraged the adoption of cobalt therapy. And both groups of states succeeded in reducing the adoption of open-heart surgery (see chapter 5).[15]

In summary, policy in the United States, both on paper and in reality, is in transition. It started with an initial, rather tentative, commitment to the concept of area planning. State certificate-of-need legislation and the national health planning law of 1974 have made that commitment considerably more serious and substantive. The application of these laws can take policy in a number of directions; the 1974 law even states that the planning agencies should weigh costs and benefits when deciding which projects to include in their plans. But in their present form, U.S. policies—like those of many other countries—are based on the belief that it should not be necessary to go beyond step 2, or perhaps just to the edge of step 3, to reduce the growth in costs to an acceptable level.

14. See Lewin and Associates, *Evaluation,* pt. 1. The computed tomography scanner, which arrived on the scene in 1973 when planning and review were reasonably well established in many areas, provides a good illustration of the difficulties (U.S. Congress, Office of Technology Assessment, *Policy Implications of the Computed Tomography (CT) Scanner* [GPO, 1978]).

15. These results are not necessarily inconsistent with the findings of Salkever and Bice that certificate-of-need laws slowed the growth in numbers of beds in those states below the rate in states without such laws but that investment per bed increased, leaving the total level of investment unaffected (David S. Salkever and Thomas W. Bice, "The Impact of Certificate-of-Need Controls on Hospital Investment," *Milbank Memorial Fund Quarterly: Health and Society,* vol. 54 [Spring 1976], pp. 185–214). If the effects of certificate-of-need reviews have, in fact, been limited to certain states and certain technologies, most hospitals in most states have still had abundant opportunities to invest in things that were not covered by the law—because their cost put them in the exempted category, or because they did not constitute a change in service for the hospital—or that were not perceived as problems by the reviewers in their states.

Sweden

The concept of regionalization as a means for promoting efficiency has influenced the health policies of many countries, but probably no country has embraced it more wholeheartedly than Sweden. In the early 1960s the national parliament approved the Engle report, a detailed proposal for regional systems of hospitals prepared by Arthur Engle, then head of the National Board of Health. This regional plan, which has since been expanded to include all medical care services, has been overlaid on a financing system in which the twenty-five county governments of Sweden own almost all the hospitals and provide most of their funds. In fact, 70 percent of all medical care costs in Sweden are paid by the counties out of the receipts from proportional income taxes.[16]

The first step in regionalization was to divide the country into a number of medical care regions—or, more specifically, hospital regions—each large enough to support a more or less self-sufficient hospital system. Engle established the size of these regions by asking physicians at teaching hospitals the optimal size for highly specialized departments such as neurosurgery (optimal in the sense that the department would be large enough to support all the research, training, and services that these physicians believed to be necessary for a good department) and the optimal ratio of specialty beds to population. This allowed him to calculate the approximate minimum population needed in a region. He then considered various possible configurations of regions in light of the amount of time it would take most people in the region to travel to a hospital, particularly a central regional hospital. The result was seven hospital regions, which ranged in size of population from 650,000 to 1.6 million in the early 1970s.

A graded series of hospitals was then defined. At the top of the pyramid are the seven regional hospitals, which provide highly specialized medical services (neurosurgery, plastic surgery, thoracic surgery, cardiology, urology, and so on) and which almost always serve as university teaching hospitals as well. County hospitals, of which there are approxi-

16. Except as noted, the information in this section comes from D. J. Beckley, "Regional Health Planning in Sweden: A Comparison," *Hospital Administration in Canada,* vol. 17 (April 1975), pp. 41–43; Ragnar Berfenstam and Ray H. Elling, "Regional Planning in Sweden: A Social and Medical Problem," *Scandinavian Review,* vol. 63 (September 1975), pp. 40–52; and Vicente Navarro, *National and Regional Health Planning in Sweden,* DHEW (NIH) 74-240 (GPO, 1974).

mately twenty-five, provide general hospital care for the surrounding population and specialty care in such things as gynecology, pediatrics, ophthalmology, and orthopedics for the entire county. At the bottom of the hospital pyramid are over fifty district hospitals (fifty-three in the early 1970s), and these provide the basics—general surgery, internal medicine, anesthesiology, and diagnostic X-ray—for about 75,000 or 100,000 people. Basic though they are, district hospitals are not necessarily small, and may have 500 beds or more. Below this last level of hospital is the local health center, which may include a nursing home or some other facility for long-term care.

The goals of the regional system are to emphasize preventive care, outpatient care, and care at home, and—most particularly—to make sure that hospital facilities are used as efficiently and intensively as possible. Only the capacity that can be fully used is supposed to be provided at each level of hospital care. For each level, the services to be offered and the ratio of beds to population are spelled out; apparently even the different numbers of staff per bed and the proportion of beds that should have each number are spelled out in some detail. This is done to avoid underuse and "unnecessary" duplication of facilities, and if a patient needs a higher level of care than is available at his local hospital, he is supposed to be transferred to the nearest hospital in his region that does provide the care he needs. The regional plan is not aimed at controlling the distribution of technologies directly, but the limitation of specialized departments clearly affects their distribution.

In short, the system is an elaborate intervention on behalf of technical efficiency—keeping the costs of services down without questioning the level of services to be provided. That this is the aim of the system is underlined by the method of projecting demand: essentially, demand is estimated by projecting past trends, and adding something extra if it is thought that certain needs or population groups were neglected in the past. It is not always possible to provide the full measure of resources necessary to meet the projected use right away, but that is the goal and failure to achieve it is temporary and unavoidable, rather than permanent and intentional.

The efficiency approach is refined still further by the activities of SPRI, the Swedish Planning and Rationalization Institute of the Health and Social Services, established cooperatively by the national and county governments in 1968. The work of the institute is to help promote planning and coordination, to collect information that would help in planning, and to develop norms and standards for medical buildings and standard specifications for hospital equipment. The types of study published by SPRI reflect the emphasis on efficiency: designs for diagnostic X-ray departments, the layout and organization of intensive care units, tests of disposable dialyzers, and so on.[17]

The extent to which the regional plan has been put into practice is not clear, but everyone seems to agree that practice does not yet match principle. Application of the plan is voluntary and depends on the cooperation of the twenty-five county governments. One article describes regionalization as "now in an advanced planning stage,"[18] while other sources express varying degrees of doubt about how completely it has been accepted.

There are bits and pieces of evidence to suggest the extent to which practice and principle diverge. In view of the rhetoric about de-emphasizing hospital care—rhetoric which has surely by now been used countless times in every industrialized country—the most striking fact is the unusually heavy emphasis on hospital care in the Swedish system. In 1968 in all types of hospitals, there were sixteen beds per 1,000 people in Sweden, eight in the United States, and ten in England.[19] Patient days in general hospitals per 1,000 population were 1,569 in Sweden, 1,154 in the United States, and 1,132 in England.[20] At the same time, outpatient visits to physicians per person per year were far fewer in Sweden than in the other two countries: less than 3 in Sweden, about 4.5 in the United States, and almost 6 in England.[21]

And, of course, local pressures cause specialty departments to be established where they are not supposed to be. In the early 1970s, nineteen of the fifty-three district hospitals had specialties that were supposed to be limited to hospitals higher in the pyramid. Obstetrics-gynecology was the most frequent and was attributed to an understandable desire on the part of the populace and the hospital physicians to have the service nearby. Nor does regionalization ensure that services are always produced in

17. Swedish Planning and Rationalization Institute of the Health and Social Services, *SPRI's Publications 1975: Summaries* (Stockholm: SPRI, 1976); see also ibid. *1972, 1973,* and *1974.*

18. Berfenstam and Elling, "Regional Planning in Sweden," p. 42.

19. The data in this paragraph are from Odin W. Anderson, *Health Care: Can There Be Equity? The United States, Sweden, and England* (Wiley, 1972), pp. 122, 131, 134.

20. Most of the difference between Sweden and the United States was due to the considerably longer average stay in Sweden.

21. The Swedish government plans to double the number of doctors during the 1970s, with the aim of raising the level of outpatient visits.

optimally efficient quantities (this is probably inevitable: there is no guarantee that the optimal quantities of each service will always, or indeed ever, be consistent with the same size of hospital). A study of the costs of computed tomographic scanners reported that pneumoencephalograms and cerebral angiograms (rather specialized and dangerous neurodiagnostic tests) were done at most, if not all, hospitals in Sweden.[22] The majority of the local hospitals did far fewer than were estimated by neurological specialists as the minimum necessary to stay properly skilled in the performance of these exams.

Even though the regional plan is not yet fully in place and thus presumably not as effective as it might be, the Swedes are beginning to move toward the next step and to ask questions about benefits. SPRI has expressed an official interest in studying the outcomes of medical treatment, and a few of its studies do this. One of the most interesting followed the results of a screening program carried out in 1964 and discovered that, although many therapies were initiated or changed as a result of the screening, an extensive statistical analysis was unable to discern any advantage in health status five years later; the study concluded that screening should not be a high priority.[23] And quite recently, SPRI began a program to establish "medical care programmes" (which we would call medical protocols), an explicit documentation, disease by disease, of the indications for treatment, for surgery, and for discharge from the hospital, with particular focus on the resources used at each stage. This is a variation on the first approach to the evaluation of benefits—making professional judgments explicit. It is interesting in this regard that the United States appears to have carried this approach farther than any other country and there is currently a debate in several European countries over whether to adopt such U.S. devices as medical audit committees, utilization review, and peer review.[24]

Great Britain

Great Britain embarked on one of the world's most famous social experiments, the National Health Service, in 1948. The service is available

22. Egon Jonsson and Lars-Åke Marké, "Computer Assisted Tomography of the Head: Economic Analysis for Sweden" (Stockholm: Swedish Planning and Rationalization Institute, July 1976).

23. *SPRI's Publications 1974* (Stockholm: SPRI, 1975), p. 66.

24. Egon Jonsson, "Medical Care Programmes" (Stockholm: SPRI, October 1976).

to everyone, even foreign tourists. Little or no payment is required at the point of service and most of the financing comes from general tax revenues. The health service owns and operates most of the hospitals in the country.[25]

From the first—or at least after the first few years, when it became clear that, unlike the Marxist state, nationalized medical care would not do away with the need for itself—the health service has operated subject to the explicit policy that less than the full amount of resources demanded at zero prices would be provided. The most palpable sign that resources have been limited is the long waiting list for hospital care, which for years hovered at 500,000 people—in a nation of 50 million people—and has recently begun to increase.[26] And the policy set for the late 1970s projected that the health service budget would grow in real terms only 2.6 percent in fiscal year 1977 and 1.8 percent annually in the following years.[27]

The primary constraint facing the service, then, is the policy (which has so far survived the chorus of complaint against it) of limiting its total budget. From the total, amounts are allocated to the fourteen regional authorities, and through them to the lower authorities, until each hospital receives its own budget allocation for the year. (Under the reorganization of 1974, the new regional health authorities and the ninety area health authorities under them have responsibility for what before that time were administratively four separate services: the hospital service, the family practitioner service, local health authorities, and the school health ser-

25. Except as noted, the information in this section comes from three sources: Manuel L. English, "Budgeting for National Health Expenditure: The British System," *World Hospitals,* vol. 12 (July 1976), pp. 164–70; George E. Godber, "Decision-Making System and Structures in the British National Health Service," *Hospital Progress,* vol. 57 (March 1976), pp. 82 ff.; David Owen, "The Organisation and Management of the NHS," *Hospital and Health Services Review,* vol. 72 (July 1976), pp. 239–44.

26. "Waiting-Lists Lengthen," *Lancet,* vol. 1 (January 15, 1977), reviewed in *Medical Care Review,* vol. 34 (February 1977), pp. 188–90.

27. See Keith Barnard and Chris Ham, "The Reallocation of Resources: Parallels with Past Experience," *Lancet,* vol. 1 (June 26, 1976), pp. 1399–400; and Department of Health and Social Security, *Priorities for Health and Personal Social Services in England: A Consultative Document* (London: Her Majesty's Stationery Office, 1976), p. 1. These rates are lower than the service had been permitted in previous years and reflect both the difficulties of the British economy and the related decision to hold public spending in check and let any new growth take place only in the private sector.

vice.[28] Before 1974, only the hospital service had a regional level of administration, the regional hospital boards.) For most of the history of the service, the budget allocations to the regions and through them to the hospitals were essentially last year's allocations plus something for inflation plus perhaps 2 or 3 percent for growth and new services. Not too surprisingly, this left the regional distribution of resources much as it had been in 1948, and since 1971 the allocation process has been moving toward the use of a formula for calculating the regional shares. By the early 1980s, the formula is supposed to produce a distribution of resources that more equitably reflects the needs of the different regions.[29]

The regional authorities are reminiscent of the regional plan in Sweden, but there are some important differences: the regional authorities are not just boundary lines on a map but administrative agencies with considerable power of their own; and there is no nationally prescribed plan for them to follow. The regional authorities, and before them the regional hospital boards, are responsible for most of the important decisions about which hospital services are to be provided and in what configurations, given the constraint imposed by the budget they receive from the national Department of Health and Social Security (DHSS). According to Godber, DHSS advocates, encourages, and even offers financial inducements to promote certain policies, but it does not command; this guidance "is most precise in the financial and medical manpower fields and less so in questions of service priorities."[30]

28. The ninety areas are further divided into 200 districts, with an average population of 250,000. Essentially, district boundaries are defined in terms of hospital catchment areas. The fourteen regional authorities, ninety area health authorities, and 200 districts are in England. In Wales and Scotland (and Northern Ireland) the regional functions are handled by the central national department in each country and there is no separate regional level of administration.

29. The formulas were redesigned by the Resource Allocation Working Party, which published its report in 1976 (*Sharing Resources for Health in England: Report of the Resource Allocation Working Party,* Department of Health and Social Security [London: Her Majesty's Stationery Office, 1976]). Allocations are made separately for operating expenses and capital investment and cover all the health and personal social services managed by the regional authorities. Each formula begins with the population of the region—the most recent actual head count for operating expenses and a projection five years ahead for capital; the part of the formula having to do with general inpatient hospital care then weights the population by national use rates for the different age and sex groups and by standardized mortality and fertility rates.

30. Godber, "Decision-Making System," p. 94.

Clearly then, there is some scope for regional discretion and for regional differences in approach and in result. This probably explains why there is no account of national policies or national trends related to the regulation of medical technologies—and with the overall budget constraint, perhaps there is no need for any. In any event, it is the regional authorities who are primarily responsible for weighing the alternatives and deciding what will be provided and what will not. They have detailed control over the development of health manpower, especially hospital manpower. They are responsible for developing long-term plans for capital investment and for overseeing their execution. And coming even closer to decisions of direct relevance to the distribution of medical technologies, they are responsible for deciding which specialties should be offered in which hospitals of the region. It is not clear to what extent some of these decisions may be delegated to the area health authorities.

From time to time, decisions about particular technologies do get made at the national level. Godber relates that the use of dialysis for chronic kidney failure began at a few major medical centers, and when it became clear that dialysis was ready to spread beyond these enclaves, a national conference was held to consider alternative policies. The conference recommended that regional centers be established. DHSS obtained a special allotment of funds, and with the advice of an expert committee that grew out of the conference, distributed grants to regions that submitted acceptable plans for dialysis centers. Godber observes that "such allocation is an unusually explicit example of national, regional, and local planning."[31] The case of coronary care units is apparently more typical. There, a national conference resulted in guidelines to be used at the discretion of regional and local planners.

Screening programs appear to have been the object of national, as opposed to regional, policies much more frequently, perhaps because they cross the boundaries of the (until 1974) four distinct health services. National screening programs for cervical cancer and phenylketonuria were developed with the advice of a national committee, the Standing Medical Advisory Committee. A screening program for raised intraocular pressure, a sign of potential glaucoma, was considered and rejected on the committee's advice; interestingly, the results of a controlled trial of such a program by DHSS were taken into account in this decision.

The British system clearly goes farther than any of the four, and possi-

31. Ibid., p. 86.

bly farther than any other country, in making judgments about benefits and in choosing explicitly to limit resources to a point that falls short of providing every service that might be beneficial. The primary decision, to limit the overall budget of the National Health Service, is effectively a policy about the benefits of medical care in general, rather than the result of separate consideration of the costs and benefits of all the possible services that could be provided. But some of the decisions are specific—the screening programs, for example. And in the case of renal dialysis, the level of resources provided specially for that technology has lagged behind the level necessary to provide dialysis to everyone who could possibly benefit from it, and behind the levels provided in other European countries and in the United States.[32]

Possibly as a result of its firm policy against interfering in clinical decisions, beyond the setting of broad resource constraints, Britain has not developed a systematic program of testing the benefits of medical practice, and particularly new technologies, although it would seem to have more reason than any other country to consider such tests useful. It has apparently not even made full use of the studies that are available. The provocative study by Mather and his colleagues,[33] which compared intensive care and home care for heart-attack patients, is apparently as much without honor in its native land as elsewhere.[34] But their value is officially recognized. The Cogwheel reports noted the dearth of outcome studies and their great potential usefulness, and, in Godber's words, "urged more general pursuit of such studies."[35]

France

France is unique among the four countries, and would probably remain unique even if a larger number of countries were considered. As a con-

32. S. L. Dombey, D. Sagar, and M. S. Knapp, "Chronic Renal Failure in Nottingham and Requirements for Dialysis and Transplant Facilities," *British Medical Journal*, vol. 2 (May 31, 1975), pp. 484–85.

33. H. G. Mather and others, "Myocardial Infarction: A Comparison Between Home and Hospital Care for Patients," *British Medical Journal*, vol. 1 (April 17, 1976), pp. 925–29.

34. Willis J. Elwood, "Longer Term Perspectives of the NHS: Some Reflections Arising from the Manchester Seminar," *Hospital and Health Services Review*, vol. 71 (December 1975), p. 425.

35. Godber, "Decision-Making System," p. 94.

sequence of the hospital reform act of December 31, 1970, the French have developed a detailed system of regulation aimed explicitly and directly at controlling the adoption of medical technologies. The system involves a list of technologies for which approval is required, indexes of need in the form of equipment-to-population ratios prescribed by the national Ministry of Health, and, as a crucial step in the consideration of requests, the development of a map for each technology showing the numbers and locations of equipment in place, equipment authorized but not yet in place, and proposed new installations.[36]

The law applies to all institutions involved in providing medical care, whether or not they provide hospitalization.[37] Responsibility for approving requests depends on which technology is requested. Unless authority is specifically claimed by the Ministry of Health, the regional prefects make the decisions after receiving the advice of their regional hospital commissions. But in fact the Ministry of Health has claimed authority for most of the technologies on the list, on the grounds that their distribution can only be properly viewed from the national, or at least multiregional, perspective. The minister makes his decisions with the aid of the maps supplied by the regions and the advice of the National Hospital Commission.

The initial list of items subject to approval was published on November 30, 1972. Eight items were listed: autoanalyzers (laboratory equipment capable of doing a variety of tests automatically); heart-lung machines; hyperbaric chambers; linear accelerators capable of emitting more than 500 kilovolts (kV); cobalt radiotherapy; scintillation cameras; radioisotope scanners; and artificial kidneys. The decree ended with a general clause stating that approval is required for any piece of equipment with a purchase price of 150,000 francs or more, or a monthly rental and maintenance cost of 5,000 francs or more.

Two more items were officially added to the list in September 1975:

36. This section is based on a series of circulars and decrees published in French by the Ministry of Health to spell out the procedures to be used under the new law— for example, the list of equipment to which it applies and the methods to be used in preparing the maps. Specifically, these are decrees no. 72-1068 of November 30, 1972, and no. 75-883 of September 23, 1975, and the following circulars: no. 85 of February 26, 1973, nos. 260 and 261 of July 16, 1973, an unnumbered circular of August 1973, no. 204 of June 12, 1974, no. 495 PC 2 of June 15, 1976, no. 530 of November 3, 1975, and no. 381 of May 6, 1976.

37. The approval process apparently differs in some respects for private and public institutions, but none of the circulars or decrees describes the differences.

the laser photocoagulator and the computed tomography (CT) scanner. The addition was primarily a formal one for the CT scanner since, unlike the photocoagulator, it had been subject to the regulations all along because it fell in the class of items covered by the general clause based on purchase price.

Regardless of who is responsible for the final decision, the minister hands down the indexes of need on which the decision should be based. How the minister arrives at these equipment-to-population ratios is only hinted at in the circulars. He clearly seeks the advice of that part of the medical community expert in the uses of the technology, but what information they use in arriving at their recommendations is never described, either in general or for a particular case. Clearly, they can take into account the results of randomized controlled trials, or other studies of efficacy, but it is impossible to say whether they do. And in theory, the approval process could stimulate a program of clinical trials aimed at investigating the costs and benefits of the technology for different types of patients. But this is nowhere stated to be the intent of the law or of the regulations.

In the absence of evidence to the contrary, it seems likely that the equipment-to-population ratios are aimed at achieving the efficiency goals of the second step of the hierarchy: keeping the costs of providing whatever is provided to a minimum, while leaving the questions of benefits and how much should be provided out of the deliberations. To the extent that questions about benefits are asked explicitly, the approach appears to be that of the first tentative move to step 3 of the hierarchy: making the judgment of the medical profession explicit, and collective, through the medium of the expert committee, rather than leaving the answers entirely to the judgment of individual practitioners.

As of March 1978, equipment-to-population ratios had been prescribed for only six of the ten listed technologies. They are generally published in conjunction with reports and directions concerning that technology—for example, reports of the number of installations already in place in each region, or directions for the preparation of the regional maps for the technology.

Five of the ratios were published in 1973. They were:

—One hyperbaric chamber per 500,000 people.

—Thirty chronic hemodialysis stations per million people (not including dialysis units used in the home, for which approval is *not* required).

—Autoanalyzers only to be approved for laboratories whose test volume is at least two million *B* per year.[38]

—One linear accelerator per million people.

—One cobalt therapy unit per 200,000 people.

The ratio for the CT scanner (one per million people) was published in May 1976. The same ratio applies to head scanners and to the newer body scanners, but the minister stated that head scanners should be given priority for approval. He recommended that a few body scanners be approved so that French physicians could begin to gain experience with them, but that they be limited for the near future to major medical centers.[39]

Some of the difficulties of trying to arrive at these ratios are suggested by a recent change in the ratios involving linear accelerators and cobalt therapy units. Before all the regions had finished preparing maps based on the first ratios, the specialists whose opinions had formed the basis for the ratios changed their minds. They decided that linear accelerators should not be treated as an undifferentiated group, but divided into those capable of ten million volts (MV) or less (which have much in common with cobalt in terms of their therapeutic properties) and those capable of more than ten MV. The new ratios are one linear accelerator of more than ten MV per million people, and one cobalt therapy unit *or* one linear accelerator of ten MV or less, for every 200,000 people. The change has created some obvious possibilities for maneuver. While the total number of very high energy accelerators in France at the time the circular was published, fifty-two, was precisely one for every one million people, three regions were without such an accelerator. Similarly, while the number of cobalt units plus accelerators of ten MV or less (274) exceeded the number needed nationally based on the ratio (263), some areas could still qualify as needing additional units. Further, accelerators were accepted as having some therapeutic advantages over cobalt so that, in spite of the fact that accelerators cost more, the ministry indicated that it would be

38. *B* is a unit of relative value, or complexity, designed by the Ministry of Health to reduce different lab tests to a common measure that can then be added. For example, a test for sugar in urine is assigned a value of 2 *B*, a test for immunity using immunoelectrophoresis a value of 120 *B*.

39. As of August 1976, there were 1.5 CT scanners of both types per million population in the United States. Adding the number of scanners on order brought the ratio to three scanners per million population (U.S. Office of Technology Assessment, *Policy Implications of the Computed Tomography (CT) Scanner*), p. 52.

inclined to approve requests to replace existing cobalt units with accelerators.

The discussion in this section is limited to medical technologies, narrowly defined in terms of specific kinds of equipment, but the system apparently applies to a wider range of medical care resources, in particular the distribution of specialty departments. The circulars reviewed refer in passing to other circulars setting out the steps followed in developing maps for departments of medicine, surgery, obstetrics-gynecology, and neurosurgery. Apparently, the same process of ratios and maps applies. The French system is clearly a variation on the theme of regionalization and its overlap with other variations on that theme is made more obvious by the inclusion of specialty departments.

Conclusions

The introductory section of this chapter describes a hierarchy of steps that governments might go through as they move from their initial policy that everything of benefit can and should be provided, to a growing appreciation of the infinity of good things that are possible in medical care. Of the four countries discussed in this chapter, three—the United States, Sweden, and France—have so far limited themselves to the early steps, still hopeful that everything of real benefit can be done if only it is done with maximum efficiency (step 2) and if care is taken to make sure that nothing is done that is without any benefit whatsoever (step 3). Scattered evidence suggests that these three countries are representative of a larger number.[40]

Certainly resources will be better used if technical efficiency can be improved and worthless procedures abandoned, but the number of uses for resources in medical care is still virtually infinite. Some uses stand out because they require so many resources for so few people: modern care for serious burns saves people who would not survive without it, but it does so at enormous expense; the annual cost of renal dialysis, even at

40. For example, West Germany and the Netherlands passed new laws having to do with capital investment and planning for medical care in the early 1970s. See *Cost and Utilization Control Mechanisms in Several European Health Care Systems,* Report by the Staff to the Senate Committee on Finance, 94 Cong. 2 sess. (GPO, 1976).

home, is higher than the income required to put a family of four above the poverty line. There are numerous other, less obvious, ways to use resources as well. For example, people in medical care can be trained and retrained in a continual attempt to insure that someone with just the right knowledge is there when the patient needs him.

If the preceding view is correct, then governments, and more generally the societies they represent, will be forced to step 4 of the hierarchy, back to a variation of the question they had hoped to avoid by moving from an ordinary market for medical care toward complete third party coverage, Is it beneficial *enough*? Controlling costs means deciding that some things, although beneficial, are *not* beneficial enough. And that means that resources, and therefore medical services, must somehow be rationed.

The possible approaches to rationing can be characterized by describing the two extremes. One extreme is to limit the total resources available for medical care without making any judgments about particular kinds of care. For example, as in Britain, the total budget for medical care could be set at less than the amount needed to satisfy the demands of patients and providers at zero prices and rationing could then be achieved by queuing. Or a flat coinsurance rate that is the same for all kinds of medical care (but that might be different for different income classes) could be set, and patients and doctors would decide whether—considering the expense to the patient—a particular service was worthwhile.[41] In either case, the questions of which particular technologies to invest in and who would get to use them would be answered by the aggregate results of many individual decisions, not by the government, although a general and not necessarily very accurate sense of benefits and costs at the margin would probably influence the decision about the level of the total budget or the coinsurance rate.

At the opposite extreme, the government could make decisions about each technology individually, based on that technology's costs and benefits. The decisions would specify whether it should be provided at all, at what level, where, and to what kinds of patients. One proposal of this type would allow only services that have been proven beneficial (potentially, beneficial enough) to be provided free at the point of service under a national health insurance plan; the patient would have to pay the full cost of any others. Certificate-of-need review also falls in this category,

41. Coinsurance, or the coinsurance rate, refers to the percentage of the cost the patient must pay. For example, under Medicare the patient is responsible for 20 percent of the cost of all doctors' services after the first $60 worth each year.

as do the professional standards review organizations (set up by the Social Security Amendments of 1972), which review the need for hospitalization under the Medicare and Medicaid programs.

The second approach, judging technologies one by one, requires a great deal of information that the first, in its pure form, does not. The decisions about how many resources to devote to each quite obviously depend on knowing what the costs and benefits of each technology are. (In the first approach, this information is nice but not necessary. Better decisions can be made about the use of resources if it is available, but no matter how bad individual decisions are, resources will be limited.) Whoever makes the case-by-case decisions needs to know whether the technology benefits anyone at all, how great its benefits are for different kinds of patients if it has benefits, and the costs for those patients; costs and benefits must be linked and they must be broken down in enough detail to make it possible to choose among different levels of investment in a technology—an all-or-nothing approach is too crude to be very useful. Finally, the results must be trustworthy. They must be based on enough hospitals or practitioners—of the kinds likely to use the technology in practice—that whoever must make the decisions can feel reasonably confident about their truth.

In practice, the best system is almost certainly a mixture of the two approaches, with the exact proportions determined partly by the desirability of balancing the rather arbitrary nature of the first approach against the heavy information requirements of the second. It is clearly not worthwhile to engage in an expensive process of testing and decisionmaking for every technology. Which ones were worth individual consideration would depend on how expensive the technology itself was likely to be, how many people it was potentially useful for, and even some a priori guesses about the likely size of the benefits. For the others, leaving patients and doctors free to engage in trial and error—as they often do now—subject to the general constraints on their ability to claim resources, would be the most practical thing. Both in deciding how many more resources to devote to medical care and in deciding how many resources to devote to deciding about medical care, we have to ask, Given the finite resources available to the economy, is this beneficial *enough*?

chapter seven **Summary and Conclusions**

The unprecedented growth in recent years of medical care costs, and of hospital costs in particular, has been due largely to the enormous amount of resources drawn into medical care.[1] Many of the added resources take the form of new technologies, such as intensive care and open-heart surgery. The major purpose of this study has been to follow this particular strand in the growth of resources, to discover what the resources are being used for and what is being gained in return, and to illustrate more clearly than any aggregate statistics can the nature of the cost problem.

The growth of resources, hence of costs, has been made possible by the parallel growth in third party payment. In 1950, private insurance paid less than half of all hospital costs. Today, payments by private insurance and public programs like Medicare and Medicaid average 90 percent of hospital costs. Because the patient pays little or nothing directly for hospital care, he and his doctor can make decisions without worrying about cost; they do not have to ask themselves whether the probable outcome of their next move warrants the claim on the economy's limited resources, only whether there is some chance of real benefit. Third party payment puts into practice the philosophy that no one should have to think about cost when his life or health are involved.

But as doctors and patients have pursued the infinite number of good things that can be done, we have begun to understand more clearly the implications of this philosophy. For all practical purposes, there is no end to the amount of resources that can be absorbed by medical care when the economic constraints are removed. Under the pressure of rapidly rising costs, we may be ready to consider modifying the philosophy, to agree that some benefits are too small or too costly. Viewed from this perspective, the study has had a second purpose: It begins to ask and to

1. See the statistics presented in chapter 1.

156

answer the kinds of questions that need to be asked and answered if we are to deal with the issues central to the cost problem. What are we spending for particular technologies? What are the benefits? What are the possible ways to reintroduce limits on the resources available for medical care? What factors have influenced technological diffusion in the past and might offer ways to influence it differently in the future?

The Evidence from the Case Studies

Following the economic reasoning briefly set out in the preceding paragraphs, one would expect to find that as third party payment rose to its current high level—reducing the cost of care to those who make the decisions about it to near-zero or zero—growing amounts of resources were invested in care whose benefits are small relative to its costs. Under complete third party payment, investment would proceed until the marginal benefit of any further investment equaled the marginal cost, zero.

This pattern appears repeatedly in the case studies and, by its repetition, confirms the importance of third party payment for the growth of costs in general and the diffusion of technologies in particular. Intensive care accounts for 5 percent of the beds in community hospitals, more than 15 percent of their costs, and is still growing. Yet those studies that have found benefits, and many have not, suggest that these benefits are of a much lower order of magnitude than the costs. The value of many forms of respiratory therapy has been seriously questioned, and the available evidence supports the questioners. Yet respiratory therapy has spread with astonishing speed. In ways that reflect the individual nature of each technology, the pattern appears again for cobalt therapy, open-heart surgery, and, perhaps to a lesser extent, the diagnostic use of radioisotopes.

Perhaps the most probing example is renal dialysis. The number of people per million population considered suitable for long-term dialysis has nearly doubled in ten years. The old criteria excluded the very young, the elderly, and those with serious diseases other than kidney failure; the new do not. With Medicare paying the bill, the vast majority of patients receive dialysis in outpatient centers rather than at home, which relieves their families of a heavy responsibility but costs the taxpayer much more. Renal dialysis is a particularly probing example because it is probably hardest in this case to dismiss a small benefit as no benefit. Terminally ill people may not gain as much in length and quality of life as healthier dialysis patients, but it is hard to say that they gain nothing. Again, this is the crux of the cost problem: that to pursue every possible gain in medical care, however small or expensive, is enormously, perhaps infinitely, costly.

In addition to this major theme, the case studies contribute to several of the minor themes of the study. They provide an overview of some of the major changes that have taken place in hospital care over the last three decades and thus help answer the fundamental question, What is all the money being spent for? And, taken individually, they sketch out the relative costs and benefits, and the nature of those costs and benefits, for a number of technologies that are important to modern hospital care.

The Evidence from the Statistical Analyses

The statistical portion of the study investigated the reasons behind the adoption of particular technologies by individual hospitals. The possible reasons include, of course, differences in the objectives of the hospitals, but also differences in their constraints—the structure of the local hospital market, the availability of financing, and government regulation.

Two sets of data, developed from the surveys of the American Hospital Association, were used. The factors contributing to the 1975 levels of intensive care beds and of the three prestige technologies (cobalt therapy, open-heart surgery, and renal dialysis) were examined for 2,772 metropolitan hospitals. Analyses were also done of the speed of diffusion of four technologies (intensive care, respiratory therapy, the diagnostic use of radioisotopes, and the electroencephalograph) using subsets of metropolitan hospitals selected from the surveys for the fifteen-year period, 1961 through 1975. Although the same explanatory factors, by and large, were used in each of the separate analyses, the results were not compared in the preceding chapters but are reviewed and compared in this section.[2]

The scale of a hospital's activities, approximated by the number of beds in it, was uniformly important to the diffusion of these technologies. Large hospitals adopted a given technology sooner, on average, than small hospitals, and were more likely to have one of the prestige tech-

2. Because the regressions for respiratory therapy and renal dialysis were not particularly successful—the former as a result of the limited number of years respiratory therapy was included in the AHA surveys, the latter for several possible reasons discussed in the technical note to chapter 5—they are given less weight than the others, and are often ignored, in the review.

nologies. Similarly, the percentage of beds allocated to intensive care was greater for hospitals of 100 beds or more than for those with fewer beds; but here the magnitude of the difference tapered off with increasing scale. As explained in chapter 3, this pattern is consistent with the minimum size and configuration of units considered to be desirable.

Once size was taken into account, the differences between profit hospitals and private nonprofit hospitals were fairly limited. Hospitals operated for profit were somewhat slower to adopt intensive care and diagnostic radioisotopes and, as of 1975, allocated a slightly smaller percentage of total beds to intensive care; but otherwise they were as quick to adopt, and as likely to have the prestige technologies, as nonprofit hospitals of the same size. The differences between state and local government hospitals and private nonprofit hospitals were somewhat greater and more frequent. Specialized hospitals (children's hospitals, maternity hospitals, rehabilitation hospitals, and the like) were almost always slower to adopt a technology than general service hospitals or were less likely to have it at all, and committed a substantially lower percentage of beds to intensive care.

It is not surprising that involvement in teaching and research has been an important influence on technological diffusion. What is more interesting here are the differences between technologies in the importance of these activities. In every case but one, the technology was more likely to be adopted or was adopted sooner by hospitals with residency programs. The exception is intensive care; the number of intensive care beds was affected only by the largest residency programs, while hospitals with small residency programs allocated slightly fewer beds to intensive care than hospitals with no residency programs. The influence of medical school affiliation in promoting diffusion was nearly as general; only the electroencephalograph was unaffected.

But the effects of varying degrees of commitment to research, over and above any common level that may be associated with medical school affiliation, were limited to two of the technologies, intensive care and diagnostic radioisotopes. This outcome is consistent with the nature of the technologies, both of which are widely used but, at the same time, scientifically prestigious. Diagnostic radioisotopes were adopted faster the higher the level of research grants to hospitals, while the number of intensive care beds was measurably affected only by very high levels of research spending.

These results point up, and attach magnitudes to, some of the indirect effects of national policies toward medical education and research. It has always been obvious, for example, that federal support of medical research multiplies the number of new technologies available for adoption, but clearly it also influences the level of adoption. Other federal policies over the last dozen years have promoted the building of new medical schools and the rapid expansion of medical school classes. Not only are more hospitals now affiliated with medical schools and helping to train more undergraduate students, but, as the students have graduated, the number of residents in training has grown as well. Here again, the analysis attaches numbers to some of the less obvious costs of educating doctors, and the numbers can be quite large. Open-heart surgery is a striking example: medical school affiliation and an extensive program of residency training raised the probability that a hospital would adopt open-heart surgery by 0.6.[3] Few other factors even approached such importance.

The results for the incidence of disease, and the translation of disease into hospital admissions through the agency of doctors, do not suggest that these have had major effects on the diffusion of technologies. In areas with the fewest doctors relative to hospital capacity, hospitals were less likely to adopt open-heart surgery (although they were more likely to adopt cobalt therapy) and allocated fewer beds to intensive care; but the abundance or scarcity of doctors apparently had no effect on the speed with which technologies were adopted. The proportion of doctors in different specialties was important only for cobalt therapy and open-heart surgery, both of which were adopted more frequently in areas that had more surgeons. And only two incidence measures seemed to stimulate diffusion: diagnostic radioisotopes were adopted more quickly where the number of people per hospital bed was highest; and hospitals in areas with specially high levels of motor vehicle deaths allocated a greater percentage of their beds to intensive care.

If many technologies are not associated particularly closely with a major specialty group (for example, most doctors, regardless of specialty, have some use for intensive care), and if hospitals get their information about patients through doctors, then these are the sorts of results one would expect. Market studies are not a tradition in the hospital industry. The results for population growth fit this general hypothesis. Unlike the incidence of diseases, rapid growth in the population is visible to the naked eye, without the help of doctors, epidemiologists, or even the Census Bureau. And with the exception of diagnostic radioisotopes and

3. The maximum value a probability can assume is 1.0.

respiratory therapy, every technology was adopted more quickly or in greater quantities in areas with high rates of population growth: the number of intensive care beds was greater, the prestige technologies were more frequent, and intensive care and the electroencephalograph were adopted more quickly.

The results for the traditional measure of market structure—the four-firm concentration ratio (the percentage of beds in the four largest hospitals)—match the ambivalence of the theoretical literature, which has long been unable to decide whether concentrated or unconcentrated (competitive) markets are more conducive to technological diffusion. The analysis refused to take sides, showing no relationship between concentration and diffusion except in the case of open-heart surgery: that technology was adopted more frequently in competitive markets. But the example set by nearby hospitals was important; this may reflect the competition specific to a particular technology, or the availability of local knowledge about it, or both. The more hospitals that had already adopted intensive care or the electroencephalograph, the more quickly the remaining hospitals adopted them. Similarly, hospitals adjusted their allocation of beds to intensive care in the direction of the standard set by others in the same area.[4]

Because of deficiencies in the data (see chapter 2, the section on financing), the statistical analyses were not able to add much to the demonstration of the importance of third party payment provided by the case studies. Nonetheless, the results did provide some evidence of its encouraging effect on diffusion. Both cobalt therapy and the electroencephalograph showed the expected relationships with hospital insurance: they were adopted more readily where the level of insurance was higher to start with and where it grew more rapidly over the decade; cobalt therapy was also influenced in the expected direction by Medicare. The adoption of intensive care and diagnostic radioisotopes did not show any relationship with hospital insurance, but the number of intensive care beds was significantly influenced by the share of costs paid by Medicare: the higher that share, the higher the percentage of beds allocated to intensive care. Finally, although the initial level of insurance had no effect on open-heart surgery, that technology was adopted more frequently where the growth in insurance was most rapid.

The early attempts of federal and state governments to intervene in the adoption of technologies—at first with a view to speeding it, later with

4. Diagnostic radioisotopes do not follow the pattern, and it was not possible to define an appropriate measure of this factor for the analyses of the distribution of the prestige technologies.

a view to slowing it—produced some interesting results. The history of the regional medical program suggests that intensive care was the technology most likely to have been measurably affected, and the analysis bears this out: the number of beds devoted to intensive care is moderately higher in areas where the regional programs had more money to spend.

The results for state certificate-of-need laws are particularly relevant to the current emphasis on cost control. Reflecting differences among states in the opportunities to review particular technologies and in reviewers' perceptions about which technologies are good and which bad, the results show that some of the technologies were affected in some states. In states with laws that went into effect between 1965 and 1969—New York dominates this class—certificate-of-need review held down the adoption of open-heart surgery and the allocation of beds to intensive care. In states with laws effective between 1970 and 1973, the adoption of cobalt therapy and open-heart surgery was reduced, although the latter result is statistically a bit shaky.

A study of total hospital investment by Salkever and Bice concluded that certificate-of-need laws had not succeeded in reducing investment below what it would have been without them but had redirected it, away from investment in beds and toward investment in other assets.[5] This raises the question of whether the results of the present study mean that certificate-of-need laws succeeded in imposing a net reduction in hospital costs by restraining the adoption of particular technologies or whether they further redirected investment toward technologies that were not so closely watched by the reviewers. The question cannot be answered by this analysis, but it brings out a problem inherent in any case-by-case approach to rationing resources: besides the fact that case-by-case rationing is a considerable drain on resources, it requires watching everything at once—a near impossibility—in order to be successful.

Public Policies

Chapter 6 took up the general question of how to ration resources, examining in the process the current policies of four countries—the United States, Sweden, Great Britain, and France—toward medical technologies. Of the four, only Great Britain has explicitly accepted the description of the cost problem that runs through this study and decided that

5. David S. Salkever and Thomas W. Bice, "The Impact of Certificate-of-Need Controls on Hospital Investment," *Milbank Memorial Fund Quarterly: Health and Society,* vol. 54 (Spring 1976), pp. 185–214.

it cannot and will not try to do everything that can reasonably be expected to have some benefit. From its early years, the National Health Service has operated under budgets that have made it impossible to provide everything that patients, doctors, and hospital administrators would like to have at zero prices. There are clear signs that this is the case: the waiting list for hospital admission is long; and, per million population, Great Britain has fewer people on renal dialysis than the United States or Sweden.

The other three countries, and certainly the United States, still appear to believe that it is possible to do everything of benefit as long as it is done efficiently. Their policies are phrased in the language of efficiency: avoiding unnecessary duplication, using facilities to capacity, and so on. Sweden has tried to organize its hospital care into a regional system in which only certain hospitals provide specialized services and highly specialized services are officially limited to the regional hospitals. In 1970 France introduced a law under which equipment-to-population ratios for each technology are prescribed to serve as benchmarks in the review of applications for the technology from individual hospitals. The United States expanded its planning system in 1974; among other things, every state is now required to establish a certificate-of-need review process. And the United States is considering imposing limits on the budgets of individual hospitals with the idea that this will force them to be more efficient.

There are a number of ways to limit the resources available for medical care and some of them resemble, in their formal characteristics, the policies already being pursued in these three countries (the difference lies, for example, in the level at which the equipment ratio is set, not in the fact of setting it). But, by the same token, many of them cannot succeed if we persuade ourselves that it is possible to have everything we want, that we need only eliminate inefficiency, fraud, and abuse. Instead we must begin by accepting the true nature of the cost problem. If we do not, if we are determined to have everything, we will end up paying for everything, no matter what regulatory mechanisms we put in our way to complicate the process.

Once we decide that costs are rising too fast and that, in order to slow them, we are willing to modify the philosophy that cost should not be a consideration in medical care, the next question is, How do we want to accomplish the rationing that must take place? The answer will and should reflect both our philosophical preferences among rationing mechanisms and the real resource costs of those mechanisms. Almost certainly, the best answer will be a mixture of policies.

The complexity and cost of a case-by-case approach to limiting resources suggests that any approach that itself uses resources rationally should start with some more general form of constraint. The two possibilities most often put forward are an aggregate limit on total resources (as through a national budget for medical care) or the partial reintroduction of prices in the form of coinsurance for all medical care (under coinsurance, the patient pays some fraction of all the costs he or she incurs; the fraction can be related to income). The choice between these two possibilities depends on such matters as whether it is considered more desirable to ration by queuing or by price or to discourage or encourage the patient's participation in the decisions about his medical care.

Even as a general constraint, neither method is likely to be sufficient by itself. Most proposals for coinsurance include the provision that there should be an upper limit, related to income, on the amount the patient must pay in a year; beyond that point, third party payment takes over completely and some other method of rationing must be used, at least for the kind of care, such as renal dialysis, that routinely involves very high costs. Similarly, in Great Britain—which has the purest example of the limited budget approach—not everything is kept under this constraint. There are private hospitals, doctors who have private practices on the side, and even private insurance, so that those willing to pay in order to "jump the queue" can do so.

But beyond this, general constraints treat all medical care equally. It may be that, in moving toward the explicit limitation of medical care resources, we would prefer not to do this. As two obvious examples, we might prefer to encourage vaccinations more than other kinds of care, or to scrutinize major new technologies closely before they are introduced. For these purposes, a case-by-case approach would be a useful complement to the more general constraints. With the general constraints in the background to limit resources in the aggregate, the more detailed approaches could be focused on those areas in which the benefits of their use outweighed the costs—and they would not be undone by people's ability to spend freely in other directions if a decision about one prevented spending there.

The study of particular technologies can help contribute to some of the case-by-case decisions about those technologies. But more important, this study has tried to contribute to a better understanding of the choices that face us, if we are serious about controlling medical care costs, and to suggest some of the considerations involved in deciding on the best policies for controlling them.

This appendix presents the percentage distributions of the 2,772 metropolitan hospitals selected from the 1975 American Hospital Association survey, by the hospital and market characteristics described in chapter 2. These hospitals are the basis for the analyses in chapter 5 and the analysis of the distribution of intensive care beds in chapter 3. The intervals shown for each characteristic correspond to those used in the analyses.

Table A-1. Distributions of Hospitals by Characteristics of Hospitals and Their Markets

Characteristic and period	Percent[a]	Characteristic and period	Percent[a]
Size, control, and service		*Teaching and research (continued)*	
Beds, 1975		*All research grants, 1962–75,*	
Under 100	25.2	*dollars per bed*	
100–199	26.7	0	8.3
200–299	18.3	1–999	21.5
300 and over	29.8	1,000–9,999	22.4
Control, 1975		10,000–19,999	31.6
Private nonprofit	68.8	20,000 and over	16.1
State and local government	16.4	*Research grants to hospitals,*	
Private, profit	14.8	*1962–75, dollars per bed*	
Service, 1975		0	26.7
General	94.6	1–99	21.6
Specialized	5.4	100–999	22.4
		1,000 and over	29.4
Teaching and research		*Patient care*	
Medical school affiliation, 1975			
Yes	22.7	*Deaths from cancer per 1,000*	
No	77.3	*beds, annual average,*	
Residents per 100 beds, 1975		*1950–69*	
0	68.4	Under 200	16.7
1–9	18.3	200–299	33.9
10–19	7.4	300–399	38.2
20 and over	6.0	400 and over	11.3

Table A-1 (*continued*)

Characteristic and period	Percent[a]	Characteristic and period	Percent[a]
Patient care (*continued*)		*Patient care* (*continued*)	
Deaths from heart disease per 1,000 beds, annual average, 1968–71		*Percent of office-based doctors in medical specialties, 1968*	
		Under 20	18.3
Under 350	9.8	20–24	42.5
350–449	15.6	25 and over	39.1
450–549	21.2	*Percent of office-based doctors in surgical specialties, 1968*	
550–649	37.3		
650 and over	16.1	Under 30	35.9
		30–34	44.7
Deaths from motor vehicle accidents per 1,000 beds, annual average, 1970–74		35 and over	19.4
		Percent of office-based doctors in other specialties, 1968	
Under 30	17.3		
30–44	41.5	Under 15	13.9
45–59	22.1	15–19	57.6
60 and over	19.2	20 and over	28.5
		Market structure	
Population per bed, 1969–70		*Percent growth in population, 1950–70*	
Under 200	21.7		
200–249	41.8	Under 35	30.7
250–299	26.4	35–59	33.8
300 and over	10.0	60 and over	35.5
		Percent growth in population, 1960–70	
Percent of population 65 years and older, 1970			
Under 10	70.6	Under 15	48.6
10 and over	29.4	15–24	25.2
		25 and over	26.3
Percent of population female, 1970		*Percent of beds committed to intensive care in other hospitals, 1975*	
Under 51	20.4	Under 2	14.4
51 and over	79.6	2–5	60.1
		6 and over	25.5
Percent of population white, 1970		*Percent of beds in four largest hospitals, 1975*	
Under 85	37.3		
85–94	40.9	Under 50	54.3
95 and over	21.8	50–79	21.2
		80–100	18.7
Office-based doctors per 1,000 beds, 1968		Market with fewer than four hospitals	5.9
Under 175	15.8		
175–249	39.9	*Hospitals in standard metropolitan statistical area, 1975*	
250 and over	44.3		
		1–3	5.5
Percent of office-based doctors in general practice, 1968		4–6	11.9
		7–10	13.7
Under 20	17.1	11–19	15.8
20–29	62.0	20 and over	53.0
30 and over	20.9		

Table A-1 (*continued*)

Characteristic and period	Percent[a]	Characteristic and period	Percent[a]
Third party payment		*Regulation* (*continued*)	
Percent of population with hospital insurance, 1963		*Regional medical program dollars per hospital, 1967–74*	
Under 65	13.7	Under 100,000	49.6
65–74	37.3	100,000 and over	50.4
75–84	22.4	*Area comprehensive health planning dollars per hospital, 1968–72*	
85 and over	26.5	0	12.3
Percent growth in hospital insurance, 1961–71		1–4,999	14.5
		5,000–14,999	51.8
Under 10	7.8	15,000 and over	21.4
10–19	41.8	*Technology*	
20–29	25.4	*Cobalt therapy, 1975*	
30 and over	24.9	Yes	23.3
Percent of costs paid by Medicare, 1971		No	76.7
		Inpatient renal dialysis, 1975	
Under 15	8.1	Yes	22.7
15–19	22.8	No	77.3
20–24	50.0	*Outpatient renal dialysis, 1975*	
25–29	14.2	Yes	17.3
30 and over	4.9	No	82.7
Regulation		*Open-heart surgery, 1975*	
		Yes	17.9
Effective year, certificate-of-need law		No	82.0
1965–69	9.6	*Intensive care, 1975*	
1970–73	47.7	Percent of beds (average, all hospitals)	5.045
1974–75 or no law	42.7		

a. The percentages are rounded. Therefore some of the numbers in chapter 2 may differ slightly from those calculated directly from this table.

appendix B Estimating Regressions When the Dependent Variable is Binary

The regressions in chapter 5 involve a binary dependent variable, that is, a dependent variable that takes on only the value zero or one. For example, a hospital does (one), or does not (zero), have a cobalt therapy facility. If this dependent variable, y, is thought to be a linear function of k explanatory variables, the relationship can be expressed by the usual regression equation:

$$(1) \qquad\qquad y_i = \alpha + X_i\beta + \varepsilon_i$$

where X_i is a $1 \times k$ row vector of explanatory variables, β is a $k \times 1$ column vector of coefficients, and i denotes the ith observation. When y is binary, predictions of y produced by equation 1 are interpreted as probabilities, and, together with the restrictions that these estimated probabilities may not be greater than one or less than zero, the equation is referred to as the linear probability model.

Two problems arise when, as in chapter 5, the method of ordinary least squares is used to estimate this model. First, ordinary least squares does not incorporate the constraints that the predictions, $\hat{y}$, can only take on values between zero and one, and thus there is nothing to prevent estimates produced by the equation from falling outside this interval. Second, when the dependent variable is binary, the error term, ε_i, is heteroscedastic, in violation of one of the assumptions on which ordinary least squares is based. In particular, if the assumption that the error term has zero mean is retained, its variance follows the form $E\varepsilon_i{}^2 = Ey_i(1 - Ey_i)$, where E is the expectations operator. Heteroscedastic error terms mean that the estimates of the coefficients β will not be as efficient, that is, their variances will not be as small, as if the error terms were homoscedastic. Further, since the error structure is nonnormal, the usual hypothesis testing procedures, which are based on an assumption of normally distributed errors, will apply only asymptotically.

Some of the alternative estimation methods that have been proposed involve transforming the probability, which must lie between zero and one, into a variable that can take on any value between minus and plus infinity, by making use of a cumulative distribution function. The probit method uses the normal cumulative distribution function for this purpose, the logit method the logistic cumulative distribution function. Other methods that have been proposed involve estimating equation 1 subject to the constraint $0 \leq \hat{y}_i \leq 1$, or using the ordinary least squares estimates to predict $\hat{y}_i$ and then estimating the equation again with each observation weighted by $\sqrt{\hat{y}_i (1 - \hat{y}_i)}$.

While each of these alternatives meets some of the criticisms of ordinary least squares, none is clearly superior to it. As a rule, they are more costly than ordinary least squares in computer time, more sensitive to specification error, and more difficult to present and explain, even to a reader with a fair degree of statistical sophistication. The last is a problem of particular importance for work intended to contribute to public discussion of the issues in medical technology.

Each of the proposed alternatives suffers as well from its own particular deficiencies.[1] For example, one variation of the logit method requires repeated observations for each value of the explanatory variable(s). If the variable is continuous and values are grouped to achieve "repetitions," with the mean of each group then used in the regression, an errors-invariables problem is introduced. As another example, Theil and Pindyck and Rubinfeld suggest that the probit transformation is theoretically inappropriate for many economic applications, although they do not suggest which applications, or why.[2] If this is the case, the problem may apply to the logit transformation as well since it is very close in form to the probit.

When the advantages and disadvantages of each method are considered —and given that the true model underlying the sample data is not known —ordinary least squares appears to be at least as good as the alternatives

1. These deficiencies are discussed in Thomas A. Domencich and Daniel McFadden, *Urban Travel Demand: A Behavioral Analysis* (American Elsevier, 1975); memoranda from Gus Haggstrom to Bill Albright on logistic regression and discriminant analysis, Rand Corporation, April 3, April 9, and April 30, 1974; Robert S. Pindyck and Daniel L. Rubinfeld, *Econometric Models and Economic Forecasts* (McGraw-Hill, 1976), chap. 8.

2. Henri Theil, *Principles of Econometrics* (Wiley, 1971), p. 632; Pindyck and Rubinfeld, *Econometric Models and Economic Forecasts*, p. 247.

for regressions with a binary dependent variable. The following paragraphs discuss the evidence for this conclusion.

Consider first the problem that, with ordinary least squares, the predicted values of y may fall outside the zero-one interval, something a true probability can never do. Pindyck and Rubinfeld rate this the more serious of the two difficulties, although they give no reasons for this opinion.

Many authors exaggerate the problem at the outset by implicitly assuming that the linear probability model requires the relationships between the dependent and explanatory variables to be strictly linear.[3] As a result, they depict the prediction problem with graphs like figure B-1, which clearly cannot represent such possibilities as that, in real life, the response to x may taper off as the probability approaches the extreme values. Figure B-1 further suggests that predictions can easily extend *far* outside the zero-one interval.

The prediction problem is just one difficulty of fitting a straight line to a (possibly) nonlinear relationship. The approximation may be fairly close over the range of interest to the investigator, or it may not be. But the important point is that there is no requirement that the functional forms used in the linear probability model be linear. All of the usual transformations can be applied to the explanatory variables in this model, and the investigator is free to try any of a number of ways of approximating the underlying relationship. In fact, when the data set is large, as it is in this study, it is easy to use very flexible functional forms like (groups of) binary variables or segmented linear approximations, even though these use more degrees of freedom than simpler, and more rigid, functional forms. These can trace an approximately linear, logit, or probit relation between the dependent and explanatory variables—or an entirely different relation. Seen in this light, the problem of inappropriate predictions can be viewed as a special case of the problem of choosing the correct functional form, with probit and logit only two of the more complex ways to deal with it.

Using flexible functional forms still cannot guarantee, of course, that no prediction will ever fall outside the zero-one interval. But there is no reason to expect any to fall outside by very much and every reason to believe that estimates that do exceed the limits can reasonably be re-

3. See, for example, Marc Nerlove and S. James Press, *Univariate and Multivariate Log-Linear and Logistic Models,* R-1306-EDA/NIH (Rand Corporation, 1973); Domencich and McFadden, *Urban Travel Demand;* and Pindyck and Rubinfeld, *Econometric Models and Economic Forecasts.*

Figure B-1.

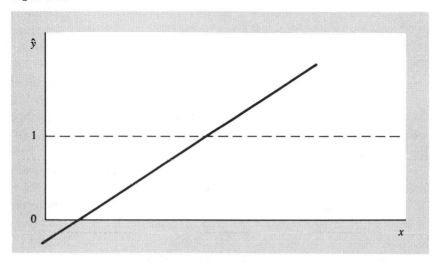

placed by 1, or 0.99, at the upper end, and 0, or 0.01, at the lower. In a study of the retention of trainees by employers, Gunderson compared the probabilities predicted by several methods, including logit and probit, and found no systematic disagreement.[4] In particular, ordinary least squares predictions that fell slightly outside the zero-one interval corresponded to logit and probit predictions that were close to the extremes of the interval. As a general rule then, it does not appear that ordinary least squares predictions either must be or are likely to be misleading.[5]

The second problem with the use of ordinary least squares when the dependent variable is binary is that the error terms are heteroscedastic and nonnormal. Thus ordinary least squares is not the most efficient estimator; that is, the coefficient estimates do not have the smallest possible variances, and the usual testing procedures—which are based on the assumption of normality—are not strictly applicable.

But for samples as large as the one used in chapter 5, the usual tests can be salvaged by referring to the asymptotic distribution of the coeffi-

4. Morley Gunderson, "Retention of Trainees: A Study with Dichotomous Dependent Variables," *Journal of Econometrics,* vol. 2 (May 1974), pp. 79–93.
5. The prediction problem can be viewed as a special case of the general problem of extrapolating. If a prediction should arise that is very far outside the interval, it could be an indication that the functional form is inappropriate or that the information in the sample is not adequate to the task. The zero-one interval can thus serve as a useful warning signal of a kind not available in most econometric applications.

cients—that is, the distribution to which they converge as the sample size grows infinitely large—rather than to their finite-sample distribution. Amemiya states that, for the linear probability model, the asymptotic distribution of the ordinary least squares coefficient estimates is normal.[6] Thus it is approximately correct to use tests based on the normal distribution when the sample is large. The mean of the distribution is the vector of true coefficients β. In the notation of this appendix, its variance-covariance matrix is $\sigma^2(X'X)^{-1}X'VX(X'X)^{-1}$, where $X = [x_{ij}]$, i denotes the observation, and j denotes the explanatory variable. V is the variance-covariance matrix of the error term.

There is little published evidence concerning the loss of efficiency associated with ordinary least squares in the presence of heteroscedasticity, and what there is indicates that it is impossible to generalize about the magnitude of that loss.[7] The magnitude depends on the particular error structure and the characteristics of the explanatory variables. But simple comparisons of the ordinary least squares variance-covariance matrix with the generalized least squares matrix—using the procedure followed by Johnston[8] and a model with one explanatory variable and the error structure usually assumed for a binary dependent variable—suggest that the efficiency loss is minor.

This is not quite the end of the difficulties. As noted earlier, the true ordinary least squares variance-covariance matrix, in the presence of heteroscedasticity, is given by $\sigma^2(X'X)^{-1}X'VX(X'X)^{-1}$. But standard regression packages incorporate the assumption that $V = I$, where I is the identity matrix, yielding the formula $\sigma^2(X'X)^{-1}$. The final question to be considered, then, is whether this conventional formula provides a reasonably accurate estimate of the true ordinary least squares variance-covariance matrix.

It is impossible to generalize about the relationship between the conventional and correct estimators. Theil analyzes the case of one explana-

6. Takeshi Amemiya, "Some Theorems in the Linear Probability Model," *International Economic Review,* vol. 18 (October 1977), pp. 645–50.

7. Goldfeld and Quandt present Monte Carlo results for a number of heteroscedastic error structures but not the one associated with a binary dependent variable. Stephen M. Goldfeld and Richard E. Quandt, *Nonlinear Methods in Econometrics* (Amsterdam: North-Holland, 1972), chap. 3.

8. J. Johnston, *Econometric Methods,* 2nd ed. (McGraw-Hill, 1972), International Student Edition, pp. 214–17. Each observation is weighted in generalized least squares. When the error terms of the unweighted specification are heteroscedastic, the weights are designed in such a way as to make them homoscedastic.

tory variable and a constant term in the presence of heteroscedasticity and concludes that the conventional ordinary least squares estimator is likely to underestimate the true variability of the estimated coefficient.[9] This will happen when large elements of $\sigma^2 V$ correspond to large absolute values of the explanatory variable. By implication, there are conditions under which the conventional formula will not be biased, but these are not discussed.[10]

A few fragments of empirical evidence suggest that, in practice, the conventional estimator will give reasonably accurate estimates of the variances of the ordinary least squares coefficients when the dependent variable is binary. Smith and Cicchetti have done some limited Monte Carlo experiments comparing ordinary least squares, with the conventional variance estimator, to generalized least squares.[11] Their results show that the variances estimated by the two methods (and the coefficients) are very close in value. Together with the simple calculations mentioned earlier, which compared the correct ordinary least squares estimator with the generalized least squares estimator, this indicates that the conventional and correct ordinary least squares estimators should produce very similar estimates.

A second piece of evidence is Haggstrom's comparison of the conventional ordinary least squares estimator and the maximum likelihood estimator of the logit transformation for regressions with binary dependent variables. Here, too, both variances and coefficients are very similar.[12] This evidence does not bear directly on the comparison of interest, but it suggests the general result that estimators that appear to differ greatly in theory may not differ much in practice.

Finally, Mohan has undertaken a Monte Carlo study of equations with binary dependent variables in which he compares ordinary least squares with other estimators under a variety of conditions: properly and improperly specified models, different degrees of multicollinearity among

9. Theil, *Principles of Econometrics*, p. 248.

10. In the case of a different sort of deviation from the assumption that $V = I$, that of autocorrelated error terms, Johnston explicitly notes one condition under which the conventional formula will not be biased. In the case of one explanatory variable, it will not be biased if the explanatory variable itself is not autocorrelated. Johnston, *Econometric Methods*, pp. 247–48.

11. V. Kerry Smith and Charles J. Cicchetti, "Some Sampling Experiments with Two Estimators for Linear Probability Functions" (unpublished paper, Resources for the Future, Inc., n.d.).

12. The ordinary least squares coefficient vector must be multiplied by the appropriate scalar, defined by Haggstrom, before it can be compared with the maximum likelihood logit coefficient vector (Haggstrom, memoranda).

the explanatory variables, and different sample sizes.[13] Directly or indirectly, this study considers all the theoretical difficulties associated with ordinary least squares. Mohan's general conclusion is that ordinary least squares outperforms generalized least squares and maximum likelihood estimators of the probit and logit transformations. It is only slightly inferior to the likelihood function of the linear probability model. These estimates are, of course, more expensive to compute than ordinary least squares.

13. Daniel F. Mohan, "Alternative Specifications of Qualitative Dependent Variable Models: A Monte Carlo Approach" (Ph.D. dissertation, Rutgers University, 1974).

Index

Adelstein, S. James, 82n
AHA. *See* American Hospital Association
Allen, Julius W., 25
AMA. *See* American Medical Association
American Hospital Association (AHA) surveys, 5, 6, 8, 72; on EEG, 86; hospitals covered by, 9–10; on hospitals' tax-exempt bonds, 29; on ICUs, 43; on prestige technologies, 115; on radioisotopes, 80; on respiratory services, 77
American Medical Association (AMA), 18, 20
Anandiah, K. M., 69n
Anger, Hal O., 81n
Ashton, T., 104n
Astvad, K., 67n
Austen, W. Gerald, 108n
Azam, Arif, 80n, 81n, 82

Baker, James P., 77n
Barendsen, G. W., 105n
Barlow, J. S., 87n
Barnard, Keith, 146n
Barton, A. Don, 79n
Bateman, N. T., 82n
Beckley, D. J., 142n
Beck, Robert N., 81n
Belinkoff, Stanton, 74n
Bender, Merrill A., 82n
Bennett, Leslie R., 83n, 84n
Berfenstam, Ragnar, 142n, 144n
Bice, Thomas W., 141n, 162
Bicknell, William J., 140n
Blood, nuclear medicine to test, 82
Bonds, hospital tax-exempt, 29
Brain scans, 81, 82–83
Brenner, Etta Rae, 110n

Breur, K., 105n
Bucci, B. Echols, 87n
Burke, Carol S., 45n, 54n, 108n
Burton, George G., 76n, 77n
Buschke, Franz, 102n, 103n, 105

Cancer: cobalt therapy for, 13, 36, 101–02; radioisotopes to diagnose, 81
Carroll, Douglas G., 42n
Cassara, Evelyn L., 76n
CCUs. *See* Coronary care units
Certificate-of-need laws: and cost control, 162; explanation of, 38–39, 137–38; federal guidelines for, 138–39; and intensive care diffusion, 57–58, 65; and prestige technologies, 129–30; and respiratory therapy, 98; and Roemer's law, 140–41; and technology adoption, 98, 141, 154
Chazan, Joseph A., 111n
Cheney, Frederick W., Jr., 76n, 78n
Chester, A. E., 140n
CHP. *See* Comprehensive health planning
Chronic obstructive pulmonary disease (COPD), 78–79
Civetta, Joseph M., 47n
Clark, T. J. H., 42n
Cloe, L. E., 15n, 102n
Cobalt therapy, 5; benefits, 106, 157; cost, 104, 105–06; development, 103; factors influencing hospital adoption of, 125–30, 161; in France, 152; hospitals with, 99–100, 115, 118; purpose, 101–02; technologies competing with, 104–05
Cochrane, A. L., 69n, 79n, 133n
Colling, A., 69n
Collins, J. V., 42n

175